AIDS
THE LAST GREAT PLAGUE

BY
SANANDA, HATONN, ASHTAR,
NIKOLA TESLA & WALTAR RUSSELL

"dharma"

Library of Congress Cataloging-in-Publication Data

Sananda, Hatonn, Ashtar, Nikola Tesla and
Walter Russell

AIDS

THE LAST GREAT PLAGUE

ISBN 0-922356-04-1

First Edition Printed by America West Publishers, 1989

Published by

AMERICA WEST PUBLISHERS
P.O. Box 986
Tehachapi, CA. 93581
Printed in the United States of America
10 9 8 7 6 5 4 3 2 1

TABLE OF CONTENTS

CHAPTER PAGE

DEDICATION

REC. #1 SANANDA

TUESDAY, OCTOBER 24, 1989 6:58 A.M. YEAR 3, DAY 069

TO THE BROTHERHOOD OF MAN. LET HIM WHO HAS EYES TO SEE--SEE! AND, HIM WHO HAS EARS TO HEAR--HEAR! THESE WORDS WHICH NOW COME FORTH ARE PORTIONS OF THE `WORD' PROMISED UNTO YOU ONES OF EARTH HUMAN. THESE MESSAGES ARE GIVEN THAT ONES CAN CHECK WITHIN YOUR OWN REALMS, THE TRUTH THEREOF. WE ARE DEDICATED TO THE BROTHERHOOD OF MAN. YOU ONES LIMIT CREATOR AND LIMIT THE CREATION, BOTH OF WHICH HAVE NO LIMITS. JUST AS YOUR PROPHETS HAVE FORETOLD THAT A THIRD OF EARTH MAN WILL FALL TO THE PLAGUES; SO, FURTHER, IT MUST ALSO MEAN THAT TWO THIRDS SHALL BE GIVEN WHEREWITHAL TO SURVIVE--BUT YE SHALL DO OF IT YOURSELVES! THE WAY IS BEING SHOWN UNTO YOU.

I SAID UNTO YOU ALMOST TWO MILLENNIUM PAST, THAT THERE WOULD BE TERRORS, AND THERE WOULD BE GREAT SIGNS FROM THE HEAVENS. WHAT DOES THE TERM "SIGN" MEAN UNTO YOU? THE GREEK ORIGIN OF THE WORD "SIGN" MEANS A SUPERNATURAL PHENOMENON INTENDED TO POINT ITS OBSERVER TO A PROFOUND TRUTH.

WHY DO YOU ACCEPT ***MAN'S*** PRONOUNCEMENT THAT THOSE COMING FROM THE HEAVENS ARE DEMONIC? IS THIS NOT THAT WHICH THE EVIL ELEMENTS WOULD WISH YOU TO BELIEVE THAT YOU WOULD TURN UNTO THEM AND AWAY FROM GOD?

WOE BE UNTO MAN WHO CONTINUES IN HIS FALSE BELIEF AND TURNS HIS COUNTENANCE AWAY FROM GOD, FOR IN THE LATENESS OF THE HOUR HE WILL HAVE TURNED AWAY HIS TRANSPORTATION TO TRAVERSE THE HEAVENS AND BE DELIVERED UNTO THE SAFETY OF THE FATHER'S PLACES.

NO MAN SHALL BE NAGGED, FORCED, NOR SNATCHED UNTO ANYWHERE; MAN WILL ASK TO BE INCLUDED AND TURN FROM HIS EVIL WAYS, FOR NO EVIL SHALL BE BROUGHT INTO THE RADIANCE OF THE CREATOR'S CITIES. IT IS TIME, EARTH BROTHER, TO GAIN OF YOUR DIRECTIONS AND HEED THE CLARION CALL OF THESE ONES WHO GIFT YOU WITH TRUTH; FOR YOU HAVE SLEPT LONG AND EVIL HAS WARPED YOUR ABILITY TO PERCEIVE CORRECTLY WITH WISDOM. YOU CONTINUE TO CLING TO THE FOOLISHNESS OF THE `LIE' GIVEN FORTH TO TERRORIZE AND TO HOLD YOU HELPLESS IN FEAR.

THE TEACHINGS OF THOSE "RELIGIOUS" ONES WHO BRING THIS UNTRUTH UNTO YOU ARE LEADING YOU INTO THE PATH OF TOTAL ERROR. YOUR PLACES OF SAFETY ARE PREPARED AS WAS PROMISED, THY SHIPS OF EAGLES ARE GATHERED---HOW MANY OF YOU WILL HAVE "PURCHASED" YOUR TICKETS TO THE WRONG DESTINATION? SO BE IT AND SELAH, FOR THE TIME OF TRANSITION IS AT HAND, THE CLARION TRUMPET HAS SOUNDED. WHO WILL HEAR THE FINAL CALL? THOSE WHO HAVE COME IN CREATOR'S NAME AND FILL THEIR COFFERS AND LOOSE YOUR VERY SOULS INTO CONFUSION SHALL BE REAPING OF THAT WHICH THEY HAVE SOWED--OPEN YOUR EYES AND SEE THAT IT IS SO. CREATOR ASKS NAUGHT OF YOU EXCEPT THAT YOU TURN FROM THE LIE AND AGAIN UNTO TRUTH---ONLY THAT YOU ABANDON THE EVIL AND TURN UNTO THE TRUTH AND PRACTICE OF THE HARMONIOUS AND BALANCED LAWS OF THE CREATION; THOSE WHICH BALANCE AND MAINTAIN THE ORDER OF THE UNIVERSES.

I AM JMMANUEL ESU SANANDA

INTRODUCTION

REC. #1 HATONN

SUNDAY, OCTOBER 22, 1989 6:45 A.M. YEAR 3, DAY 067

AIDS, THE LAST GREAT PLAGUE---sounds rather formidable does it not? *IT MOST SURELY `IS'!*

As one of the authors of this compilation of urgent material, I am pleased that we were able to actually get the information into manuscript for many efforts have been put forth to stop its production, complete with attack upon the physical being of Dharma through the use of low-frequency bombardment. Being a representative from our dimension, she has extremely high frequency patterns. This is only to point out that as you ones who dare to work on these projects herein given forth, must well expect like bombardment. There are some dark energies who keep the "enemy" informed of who is doing what. This is why we have come through this route of totally anonymous resource. The source, however, has now been pinpointed so additional attention must be given to safety. Accidents, suicides, overdoses of drugs, organ failures and cardiac arrests are "diseases" often acquired through tampering with these "planned" projects---the latter being the most recent "disease of choice". I trust our researchers are listening very carefully.

I am going to give you some facts here in this introduction so that you have no misunderstanding of intent and seriousness of your plight. I will give introduction of myself and my colleagues and if you wish to discount our truth and presence, I suggest you attend the information most carefully prior to discarding it as foolish hoax--we are not in the hoax business. I further request that you get all the available material presented by us prior to this writing. I will request an information segment be appended at the end of this journal.

Because it is most urgent that we get rapid acceptance, I shall take the liberty of utilizing your own documentation where possible so that you can more readily relate to the content. Some truth may seep, well diluted, into public attention but most never is allowed into print. A few daring publishers who understand the massive problem print a bit of truth as they can acquire it but that is not even noted by the populace.

There will be valuable information for the research community within this document because it will obviously be ridiculed and discounted and we may not get a second chance. It is predominantly, however, directed at human citizens who are the ones in absolutely directed course into grave, grave circumstance. I can only urge each reader to disperse as many books as possible, the price shall be as low as possible, comparable to copy machine reproduction so that the information can be dispersed, hopefully, worldwide--immediately! If you are to stop this plague, it must be NOW and it must be on a worldwide basis. I plead with you to hear, accept, understand, and ACT!

I will quote one of your learned scientific workers, Michael Urban, Ph.D., who has stated it most objectively and yet will not have been read by more than a tiny handful of persons. I take liberties in utilizing portions of his material for you can relate better to him than to myself at onset.

Dr. Urban begins by saying AIDS is the most electrifying terrifying, exaggerated, hyped, misunderstood and misrepresented disease of modern time. I have wanted to take exception to one or another of these descriptive words but find that I cannot. Exaggerated might be the one controversial word for there is no way to exaggerate the situation on its own merit--but then, exaggeration has been perpetrated by the ignorant so I must leave it in the description. Further, I have well over a year of additional observation from which to work, moreso, I have the ability to see both ends of a given roadway. So be it.

LETS LOOK AT THE SITUATION

Theories regarding the origins of AIDS, a retrovirus, are abundant, ranging from the nefarious CIA/WHO/NCI conspiracy theories, to Green Monkeys, to God's wrath against the poor homosexuals, to laboratory accidents or intentional contamination of smallpox and/or Hepatitis B vaccines. Some even consider it "natural evolution". Some of these are more compelling than others, while a few require a rather remarkable ability to weave together circumstantial information into a hair-raising scenario of communist world domination through the agencies of WHO (World Health Organization) and the NCI (National Cancer Institute) and, I believe you all recognize the CIA. Well, I have no hair to be raised but it most surely would stand on end if I did have such!

The latter scenario makes for interesting perspective but actually, friends, it can do nothing except distract you from what needs to be done, at this given time. I will say that along with being deliberate, the ones at the helm also have the ability to cure it and will not allow you, as a general populace access to the apparatus. This is your problem. If you feel that your elected caretakers would not do these things unto you, then I suggest you read faster, all the books we present unto you.

You must consider the possibility of conspiracy because of your Government's abysmal history of using the American public as unwitting participants in "experiments" of dubious scientific merit. A small sampling includes the various "mind control" drug programs uncovered by the Church Committee hearings of 1975 (and that was more than a decade past)---to name a few so you can look them up to satisfy yourselves: BLUEBIRD, ARTICHOKE, CHATTER, MK-ULTRA AND MK-NAOMI . . . . The violations of your proclaimed human and civil rights revealed through those hearings should have been beyond your belief--and apparently were!

Want a "funny paper" truth? How about the big TURKEY FEATHER CAPER of 1950! Your Army carried out a program in which turkey feathers infected with cereal rust spores were released over a crop of oats to determine the feasibility of using this method to initiate a cereal rust epidemic. Also in 1950, the Navy sprayed a cloud of bacteria in San Francisco to determine air-borne dispersion patterns in biological warfare applications of this type. While the Navy claimed that the bacillus used was harmless, there was one death attributed to the exercise, and thousands of residents came down with a flu-like disease. Now, brothers, these things are all documented--TRY a book called A HIGHER FORM OF KILLING---if you can find it. Publication was stopped. If you allow of it---so will publication of this be stopped. Life or death, it is up to you.

Now understand clearly, these things above were almost a half century past. Do you believe the perpetrators have been idle in forty to fifty years?

The list of "civilian" medical experiments is very long, and includes the exposure of unknowing victims to, among other things you will recognize, Whooping cough, Pellegra, Beri-Beri, Yellow fever, the good old Plague, countless drugs and toxins, exposure to dioxin, better known as Agent Orange---any of you good buddies from Viet Nam remember that one? Do any of you remember giving permission or signing an informed consent form?

I do wish to make a point of one instance because it is notorious in its "dubious" scientific value--labeled Tuskegee Syphilis Study. This study was undertaken by your U.S. Public Health Service, the predecessor of what today you label Centers of Disease Control (CDC). Now, this one does go back beyond half a century which should certainly make my point if anything will. The study monitored the progress of untreated syphilis in 400 poor, uneducated Black men in Tuskegee, Alabama. They were never told that they had the disease, and were denied treatment until 1972, when an outraged worker stumbled onto the still-ongoing study (forty years later), and blew the whistle. In the face of nationwide condemnation of the project the renamed CDC condoned the study for being "*APPROPRIATE FOR ITS TIME*"!

Oh, you say, well the higher ups probably didn't condone such a thing--read on. The CDC director who approved continued funding for this particular project in 1969, Dr. David Spencer, (I like to give credit when earned), became the New York City Health Commissioner, and a key player in AIDS policy in the early 1980's!!!

In light of previous excesses, it appears to me and my colleagues, that one cannot just lightly dismiss the speculations of experimentation and cover-up as the mere ravings of a lunatic fringe element of citizenry. The probability would seem quite high that the AIDS virus is a mutant that was adapted for growth in human cell lines in virology laboratories---and we shall most surely point out THE FACTS unto you for your perusal.

Your own medical literature has commented on the genetic homology of the AIDS virus with the bovine leukemia virus, bovine syncytial virus, and "maedi visna", a retrovirus that is endemic to sheep. In virology circles this sort of genetic similarity is rarely considered a coincidence, and in fact several very prestigious and respected virologists have publicly stated that it is unlikely that the AIDS virus could have arisen "de novo", or "naturally". Now, even in these realms, the quite rank and vulgar jokes regarding sheep herders and cowboys does not even seem amusing for it puts holes in the theory of AIDS being a homosexual limited disease.

Further compounding the possibility that this virus might be a laboratory creation is the National Cancer Institute's (NCI) thirty year history of uncontrollable cell-line contamination. The notorious HeLa cell, a particularly virulent cancer first isolated from a cervical tumor, has contaminated virtually every experimental cancer cell culture since the early 1950's. (Uncomfortable yet?) This, friends, in face of the most stringent attempts at isolation and sterilization known to man. I point this out only to get your undivided attention and illustrate the "possibility" that the AIDS virus is another famous escapee from the test tubes of NCI. You, as a public, have no way of knowing and it would be most unlikely the perpetrators would volunteer such information to an already angry public citizenry.

Well, forget the "MONKEY THEORIES" also--all of them. Just as human was created as man and not monkey, so did the AIDS virus not spring from monkeys. It may appear quite similar but other than that there isn't any connection.

GENUINE ACCOLADES TO DR. PETER DUESBERG

Dr. Duesberg, head of the Department of Molecular Biology at the University of California, Berkeley published a paper in Cancer Research in March of 1987. It was a most articulate, persuasive and scientifically accurate demolition of the notion that the AIDS virus was in itself a pathogen of sufficient virulence to explain the constellation of symptoms that is AIDS. Did you read it? I thought not! The gist is that the so-called AIDS virus violates all of the currently accepted tenets of modern virology, including Koch's postulates, and as such could at best be considered as no more than an indicator or co-factor in sera that may cause AIDS! That is an awesome FACT which makes the remainder of the story all the more horrendous for you ones.

At first glance this would seem foolishly stupid, however, it is the recombinant mutations of the AIDS retrovirus which are the real down and dirty culprits of the death machine.

Well, a lot of most prodigious egos were threatened by this publication, which has not received any significant challenge and has not in any way been discredited, the billions of dollars that had been committed for research, not to mention jobs, reputations, pharmaceuticals, et cetera, were not being challenged by renegade scientists with impeccable credentials. Virologists who were queried about Duesberg's work responded with a variety of nonsensical replies, such as "Oh, Peter's just being his cranky self", suggesting, apparently, that a twenty-one page article with some two hundred seventy-eight references was written in a pique of tantrum and irritation.

TREATMENTS?

This is a hard one to share with you desperate ones, but I shall give you the rundown---it reads like a haphazard scatter of futile attempts to find an answer. Well, there is only one that we see as having curative value, but let me continue with history.

While all of the various and sundry debates about origin, characterization and virulence of the virus were raging, people continued to die with alarming regularity. The patient and the physician were confronted with a seemingly insoluble problem. No one knew what was going on, and conventional allopathic medicine did not seem to have an answer. This situation quickly gave rise to an alternative medicine underground which proceeded to try anything and everything as a possible remedy. Moving much more quickly than your entrenched bureaucracy of the FDA, CDC and other Government health agencies, victims of AIDS and practitioners of alternative health modalities quickly struck an alliance that gave rise to treatments that included: Azidothymidine, Dideoxycytidine, Ribavirin, Dextran Sulphate, AS-721, DNCB, Isoprinosine, Imuthiol, Aloe Vera, Monolaurin, Pentamidine, Alpha Interferon, Cyclosporin, Interleukin-2, Naltrexone, Peptide-T, Hydrogen Peroxide, Ozone, and various Homeopathics, to name just a few of the major ones. Additionally, naturopathic treatments including herbs, mushroom extracts and nutritional supplements were tried and popularized in a book you can locate, written by a Laurence Badgley but I suggest you place your funds to better use.

More off the beaten path were lipid phase of the immune response studies, acupuncture, both traditional and electro-, and the various electronic modalities such as the accuscope/Myopulse, the Indumed, the Raythera, Radionics, the Lakhovsky Multi-Wave Oscillator (of which useful versions are apparently unavailable -- so be it -- in spite of claims for the junk being carried around in briefcases).

NOW, DR. URBAN AND I PART WAYS. HE LUMPS THE "SO-CALLED RIFE FREQUENCY GENERATOR", WHICH HE FEELS DOES ENORMOUS DISCREDIT TO THE WORK OF ROYAL R. RIFE, AND HE FEELS IT SHOULD REALLY BE CALLED THE "CRANE FREQUENCY GENERATOR" TO MAINTAIN HISTORICAL ACCURACY.

WELL, I DON'T COMMENT ON THE VALIDITY OF THE JUST QUOTED STATEMENT; I DO, HOWEVER, TELL YOU THAT IT WILL BE THROUGH THE USE OF THE RIFE MICROSCOPE AND FREQUENCY SYSTEM AND THE WORKS OF ANTOINE PRIORE, THAT YOUR ANSWER WILL COME AND THIS DOCUMENT WILL POINT OUT HOW AND WHY.

FURTHER, THERE IS A SUBSTANCE IN CONCOCTION PRESENTLY THAT CAN GIVE GREAT INTERIM RELIEF IN AFFECTED UNFORTUNATES. INFORMATION WILL BE APPENDED; IT IS NOT YET RELEASED BUT I SHALL GIVE YOU INFORMATION FOR

CONTACT AND INQUIRY. ONE THING THAT MAKES IT USEFUL IS THAT ONES IN THE CREATION OF THE FABRICATION ARE DULY INFECTED WITH THE VIRUS SO THERE IS A MOST VESTED PERSONAL INTEREST IN RAPID PRODUCTION AND QUALITY RESULTS. REMISSION AND CURE ARE NOT SYNONYMOUS AND DO NOT BE MISLED, BUT THERE CAN BE SOME INTERIM PROLONGATION OF QUALITY OF EXPERIENCE WHILE YOU ONES GET YOUR ACT TOGETHER AND GET ON WITH YOUR CURE.

You will find, obviously, that the problem is outreaching and one which fully involves the human immune system. It is also recognized that in individuals who are immune suppressed, the serology tests for syphilis are useless. That is to say, the AIDS virus makes a positive identification of syphilis almost impossible. Now, don't go crazy and throw this book away for I have a point to make, please.

There have been numerous reports of AIDS patients with a KNOWN HISTORY of numerous syphilis infections having negative serology for syphilis. Further, strains of disease organisms are known to change and mutate into hardier strains to avoid annihilation. You must contemplate the probability of an epidemic of not just AIDS, but of a form of tertiary or late staging Syphilis confounded by this novel new co-factor, the AIDS virus and all its cute little recombinant retroviruses which attack the DNA of the cells and change the basic Master Cellular System.

Now, if you have a disease which could partially have a cure and you utilize that knowledge you can have much value from orthodox treatment----but remember the Alabama experiment before you cast this suggestion aside as interim help.

In your early 1970's the formulation for Penicillin was changed from an aqueous Penicillin, which has a half-life in the body of only several hours at most, to Benzathine Penicillin which has a half-life of about one week. The advantages of long-acting Penicillin are obvious, particularly in the context of an office practice.

UNFORTUNATELY, IT HAS ONLY RECENTLY BECOME CLEAR TO YOUR SCIENTIFIC COMMUNITY THAT BENZATHINE PENICILLIN HAS ONE MAJOR DRAWBACK, NAMELY: IT DOES NOT CROSS THE BLOOD-BRAIN BARRIER. THIS MEANS THAT THE TREPONEME RESPONSIBLE FOR SYPHILIS CAN FIND A SAFE HARBOR IN WHICH TO LAY DORMANT FOR MANY YEARS: THE BRAIN AND THE INSIDE OF THE EYEBALL. So what--you ask? Well, friends, you have an identical set of circumstances if I might impose a bit of correlation.

It is well known that so-called AIDS dementia is one of the early diagnostic indicators of AIDS. However, in clinical diagnosis of neurosyphilis, late-staging or tertiary syphilis, it is quite clear that one can just as easily be diagnosing AIDS. Further, and back to your good old watchdogs, the CDC concurs that the time-honored treatment protocol of a single injection of 2.4

million units of Benzathine Penicillin is NOT AN ADEQUATE TREATMENT FOR SYPHILIS! Well, no amount would be adequate for you are unable to get that type of penicillin to the problem.

Since your 1970's all treatment for that which you call Syphilis has been in dosages of subclinical effectiveness. Most of your doctors have never even seen a case of tertiary syphilis, much less treated one.

The gravity of this situation was recently underscored by a paper published in your Annals of Internal Medicine, (1987; 107:492-495) in which the authors present evidence of an AIDS patient with a Kaposi Sarcoma who tested negative for syphilis on EVERY serology test, including the "gold-standard" FTA-ABS test, which is traditionally the most sensitive test of last resort. It is a credit to the physicians involved in this study that they followed through on their suspicions regarding syphilitic involvement. Ultimately, only a skin biopsy of the Kaposi lesion combined with a very specialized Warthin-Starry silver staining technique, demonstrated the abundant presence of viable spirochetes of syphilis in the tissue. Will your average physician go to such lengths to make such a diagnosis? If they did so, would the disease be adequately treated? Probably not, for the accepted treatment cannot touch the causative organism for it is most safely tucked away beyond membrane barriers.

Why bother with this dissertation? Because if THERE IS SYPHILIS PRESENT ALONG WITH THE AIDS, THE SYPHILIS WILL GET YOU AND GETTING RID OF THE AIDS WILL DO NOTHING TO SAVE THE PATIENT IN THE LONG RUN--THEREFORE A FEW MORE CORRELATIONS, PLEASE.

Syphilis is long known to be one of the most potent of all immune suppressing diseases, so potent in fact that both Kaposi's Sarcoma and Pneumocystic carinii (Hallmarks of AIDS) were first diagnosed in syphilis patients as far back as the first half of this century! Since the AIDS patient does NOT DIE OF THE AIDS VIRUS, BUT RATHER OF OPPORTUNISTIC INFECTIONS as a result of immune suppression, it would seem to make good sense to thoroughly investigate this issue of possible syphilis. This would seem particularly true when working with the homosexual population, where the medical histories of individuals typically show a 5-10 year history of chronic inflammatory diseases, multiple incidence of syphilis, gonorrhea, hepatitis, herpes, intestinal parasites, chronic drug use (both recreational and prescription), and a host of other diseases. Please do not interpret my statements as being of bigoted nature, I look only at the statistics and recognize that, unfortunate as it may be, it is the homosexual "behavior" and not love for same gender, that causes the insane results. The type of sexual encounters and the type of bodily sharing is ultimately deadly. Moral values have no influence on opinion--facts are facts and arguing over offended feelings will not get to the source of AIDS as your last great plague if you do not do something NOW!

You see, there are exceptionally good REASONS for all the "thou shalt nots". Man puts his moral stigmata upon the words as he so chooses and makes judgments--we do not, but you are caught in such a time of change that you will either again abide by the rules of The Creation or you shall perish of your own doing. LOVE needs no physical contact to survive, therefore it is the lack of self-discipline and the physical desire that you call love, which began the real spread of your plight.

AIDS is not a homosexual disease, it is not a sexual disease and condoms will not contain the virus. So be it.

Once again, you are "People of the Lie" and if not tended instantly, you are going to lose fully half of the population of this world to this plague. It is already too late for well over a third of the people. Whole continents are in full terminal strides to extinction. I plead with you to read this information and get up and do something about your position.

We are not allowed to do more than assist in response to petitions for help and through this method; in other words, we cannot just dump the apparatus and manifested substance upon you---YOU WILL DO IT OR IT WILL NOT BE DONE! WE, AS BRINGERS OF THIS INFORMATION HAVE INFINITE COMPASSION FOR YOU ONES AND WE URGE YOU TO ALLOW THE SHARING OF OUR INPUT FOR WE COME IN LOVE AND PEACE, NOT HOSTILITY NOR MYSTICISM.

THANK YOU FOR YOUR KIND ATTENTION,

COMMANDER GYEORGOS CERES HATONN

CHAPTER 1

REC. #1, SANANDA

FRIDAY, OCTOBER 6, 1989 7:30 A.M. YEAR 3, DAY 051

Greetings in Peace, Sananda present.

Dharma, it is thus forever past and present and will be thus into what man perceives to be his "future". Man will only see what he wishes to see and that which is "convenient" and comfortable unto himself. Millions upon millions have turned away from me at this point, for I rock the boat most drastically and even though humans at the helm may be brave enough to continue the journey, ones about them will "vote" them down for security and business reasons. Few--few, ever stand with me and fewer yet, unto the end. "Right" can always be compromised in the name of good discernment. There is an error in definition--judgement by any spelling whatsoever, remains judgement.

Remember, little sparrow, that if a decision is reached on any basis whatsoever that pulls away from getting my word to the masses in the most efficient and appropriate manner, it is an Earth decision. Many have accepted the responsibility and then turn from the goal to fit the needs of human pressures about them. I am asking you to hold steady the course, Dharma, for we have worked many lifespans together and there is no returning from this pathway, for we both know how this ends.

Man wishes to believe that he can simply continue into infinity spouting words and being quite pious. When the marbles are placed into play, however, the opposition does not play a fair game. Ones wish to continue to quote my beauteous words of peace and hold to self perceived ownership of truth---nay, it is right here that my troops fail me and forsake me. They do not wish to riffle the waters or become controversial.

Shocking things are perpetrated upon you ones and you sleep on. We bring truth and you sleep on.

I am going to give you something right now that is SHOCKING and yet there will be huffing and puffing and more will withdraw from you in terror. You still have not received even the most tiny portion of the truth of your plight. The anti-Christ has all but taken you, my precious ones, and you do not wish to hear of it.

The "first-strike" has already been made against your Motherland and now is the sorting and ridding of ones the higher participants wish to annihilate. Perhaps I will do this in a format of questions for I wish you ones to ponder the response.

You think you are at cross odds with that government known as the Soviet Republic. Nay, ye have been infiltrated and have worked as a coalition for many, many of these most dangerous years while you were put into addiction and rendered helpless.

You have steadily assisted, financed and shared technology directly and indirectly with that government.

SHOCK: You have the cure for AIDS already perfected. Why do you think the subject is always pushed aside in the governmental hierarchy? It will be allowed forth after the ones deemed expendable are expended. The Russians did make the first strike with your government's full approval and total acquiescence. The AIDS virus was constructed and sent forth from your Russian sector of Berlin and financed and distributed by U.S. financing and technology through the World Health Organization. This will all be covered in The Last Great Plague, which is now in our writing.

Be most cautious of the one who speaks loudest and most publicly regarding the matter, T.B., for there is a good reason he is not physically dead. He is a much greater help to the government players as he now functions. He is mostly correct, but his physical aliveness with relatively few problems is evidence enough. Our most faithful workers remain, as Dharma, living on restructured life segments.

I will speak of your Trilateral Commission to add support to what we have given unto you ones. It is worldwide, very selective in membership and totally controlled and set forth to control the planet and its peoples (those that are left to control).

I now refer to the USTEC (The United States Trade and Economic Commission). This is a joint U.S.-Soviet organization located in your New York. It has some eight to ten full-time Soviet engineers working in the selection of the best in U.S. technology for transmission to the Soviet Union. IT IS A KGB BASE!

The intent, and very existence of this establishment, is to merge the U.S.S.R. with the United States of America. It is the ultimate plan, being played out at present, for a one world government. When that is complete, you will have forfeited ALL of your human rights unto the enemy. You are witnessing the end of political history, precious ones. You are entering a world with no code of ideals. After this is accomplished, there will be neither politics nor philosophy, just caretaking of a museum of dying human history. Oh yes, the "first-strike" has been launched.

I REPEAT, DEAR BROTHERS, YOU ARE IN THE MIDDLE OF THE ENDING TIMES AND YOU QUARREL OVER WHO WILL PUBLISH MY WORK? CAN YOU NOT SEE THAT THE VERY SURVIVAL OF A SPECIES DEPENDS UPON THE WORD GOING FORTH AND MAN OPENING HIS EYES? MY ESSENCE IS PAINED, BUT AS YOU SEEK FURTHER, DEAR ONES, YE SHALL FIND THE ONE WHO IS WAITING FOR THE TASK. EFFORTS AT BLOCKING FUNDS IS CONSTANT BUT WE WILL GET THERE, BELOVED ONES, JUST KEEP THY FAITH AND, DHARMA, I PLEAD WITH YOU TO KEEP RUNNING THY FINGERS---AS RESPONSE BEGINS TO FLOW WE

WILL DO FOLLOW-UP UPON FOLLOW-UP. WE WILL USE EVERY WILLING HAND, FOR THE DEVIL WILL LOSE SOME OF HIS WORKERS WHEN THE GAME IS UNFOLDED BY TRUTH.

UFOs? Majestic-12 documents? Oh yes, but placed in front of you that you would still believe only that which "they" want you to believe. Oh yes, "they" will want "proof" from us of these higher realms---there is no original work remaining, it is only in the uncovering for it is all in truth already brought forth upon your manifested place. We shall just be in the pulling it forth.

Oberli, you must make ones such as W.S. aware that we placed some ones in protection--not for their physical protection as being ones with us, but rather to bring forth their denials. Remove those names from the document, please. I do not want those ones accepted in truth. Your brothers from this dimension come in love and peace to my troubled lands and the LIE IS OVER! Your peoples have committed atrocious crimes against your brothers and the rewards shall be reaped in further abundance. Men are playing in greed and lust for power, acclaim and lust for money in an attempt to make fortunes from half truths and payoffs to earn their higher keep.

I remind you ones, watch who comes into thy spaces with no known means of support and yet travel widely and are "seeking their balance". Most are dupes--some quite deadly and deliberate. You see, they have already succeeded--Sister will not publish our work---that should tell you much. The ploy has succeeded and I will not bring further pain unto her weary body, for she has been my most loyal friend and scribe. The flesh is most frail, dear ones, and the enemy bombardment constant unto the very ending.

Yes, Oberli, look into the writer Gerry A. Casey, July, 1989 in Western Flyer--"UFO---The Time for Telling Has Come". You are going to find your co-workers in most strange places and unexpected ones. But a lot of housecleaning must be done before the house and doorstep are in perfection. So be it.

The drug war is less than funny in our realms and you ones had better take it seriously. There is the most focused intent to deprive you of any defense through the taking of the general citizen's weapons. This will leave you at the mercy of addicted and crazed elements who will continue to have overabundance of weapons to slay you with in most varied manners.

They will not catch or prosecute Noriega of Panama. He will uncover the Pandora's box of contracts and treaties with your government. They will kill him if they can, but thus far it has not been so easy.

The interception of all of these drugs in these past days are even more comedy non-relief. It is one cartel against another and further, the government already knows where and who runs those big warehouses. It is to show "how well we are doing" to the duped public. I am going to go back to information by Ashtar and Hatonn.

There is this unique and deadly society, called Skull and Bones. It has been referred to as the Jason Society--that was more to pull Mr. Cooper out of the baseboard than anything else so let it go. The membership is totally guarded and it is most top secret. The rituals are not ever divulged and they are most interesting---some Satanic cultists would shiver my friends.

YOUR PRESIDENT BUSH IS A HIGHLY RESPECTED MEMBER OF SKULL AND BONES.

Do you want your country, birthed in goodness under God, to bear the banner of Satan himself? Well you have it!

Oberli, you must contact A. Sutton, for he needs assistance. We can no longer work in the comfort of safety. We will shield you ones but it is time to allow those ones to know we are in fact, real, and that I am returned.

I know, beloved ones, it is all but impossible that you can believe the manipulation and truth. It is shocking and unthinkable unto your minds. It is hard to believe you are controlled even to the point that your government has given immoral aid to all of your enemies, in essence killing your own men---in Vietnam that is known and documented.

Well, while you sleep you have become enslaved. The government provides you with no shelter system from atomic warfare for they think you don't need it. The communists will do exactly what they said they would do---take you over in a peaceful manner and then bury you. They happen to have their hands full at present, but it is to allow a good show later and you will ask even more government integration and the underground work can come above ground----JUST AS PLANNED.

Oh, you are going to have eventual financial disaster. Do not be put off for the delays---be grateful unto our Father for the delays that we can get further along in our mission. It would appear that things are becoming more stable---no, it is a facade and it will all come down when your enslavers deem it most appropriate.

Remember, dear ones, I HOLD THE TRUMP CARD! SO BE IT AND SELAH. Hold closely to me, little friend, for the way is lonely and most dangerous. Please remember that we do not do haphazard work either and it is so written that these things would come to pass.

Yes, it brings great pain to me to find ones who openly defraud their fellow man, to continue to speak in my name and claim he gives forth but mine truth. But man can only be fooled for a while and then perhaps he will open his eyes. It is all to mislead you of truth and I see that you can see the tangled web that has been woven to entrap you. I also see that it is almost more than you can bear---well, together we shall bear of it, for it is given that man will be allowed to know truth in these final days.

Go forth this day in peace for I see you withdrawing and moving into isolation. This is good and negative. Good, for you must take exceptional care and caution; negative, for I see you enclose your emotions which are bursting within your mind. Unfortunately for mankind, it is not you that has gone mad---SATAN PREVAILS FOR THIS IS HIS TIME.

We shall neither cease to write nor will we soften the story--truth is truth and no man shall withhold this truth from the masses for it is ordained that it shall be thus. The world shall have a chance because you ones have walked this way and, Dharma, though it seems you walk alone, others of mine also feel alone, ye are not---precious chela, ye need of no other friend, save me.

Thy dearest brothers and sisters cannot yet pull away from the tug of human bombardment and misperceptions of actions against the Laws of The Creation and God; most still are trying to re-write them to be pleasing. NO--THEY ARE HARD AND THEY ARE ABSOLUTE AND IF OUR BROTHERS FALL TO THE WAYSIDE, WE SHALL ALLOW THEM THAT, BUT WE SHALL PRESS ON AND WE WILL DO THE WHOLE OF IT IF THAT IS ULTIMATELY REQUIRED. OUR WORK MUST GO FORTH--THE MESSAGES BROUGHT FORTH IN THESE PAST BRIEF DAYS MUST GO FORTH. THE TRUTH LIES BARE IN THE EYES OF MAN IF YOU GET IT OUT TIMELY, FOR NO AUTHOR COULD PRODUCE THIS QUANTITY OF CRITICAL INFORMATION FROM HUMAN STANDPOINT. YOU WILL HAVE LOST YOUR ADVANTAGE IF DELAYS ARE ALLOWED ON PRINTING AND PUBLICATION. YOU ARE NOW WEEKS BEHIND BECAUSE OF THE PRINTING OF SPACE-GATE NOT BEING FINISHED AND I AM MOST DISPLEASED. SO BE IT.

I take my stand by thy side that you can gather of your things to go into the city. Dharma, go unto thy market and I will allow of you time to stitch some swaddle wraps for our babe who is only a few short weeks yet in the finishing--it shall be a most special child. I am sorry that ye have not been allowed the female joys of thy journey, but you will see that your little ones came forth this route to serve in their own space when the time is appropriate. I bless you ones of mine own for thy way has been so hard and I am in such humble service unto you. I place my benediction and blessings upon thy soul that you will be coming shortly into thy rightful inheritance.

I AM IMMANUEL OF GOD, I AM SANANDA

CHAPTER 2

REC. #1, HATONN

TUESDAY, OCTOBER 10, 1989 6:00 A.M. YEAR 3, DAY 055

Hatonn present, Dharma, in the Service of the Radiant One; ready to transmit and respond. I appreciate your joining me in the primary hours of this day and coming forth to pen before the dawn. It is most urgent, chela, most urgent that the information go forth--your populace is in grave circumstance. There will be no information given forth that you will truly understand, chela, but ones of intent will recognize much of incredible value. You will please not tarry over the presentations; just write, 'tis for those intended ones to receive and recognize---we will not place you in any more drastic danger. Those ones will go unnamed in this preliminary scribing. Honor unto you ones who have dared, risked and especially unto those ones who have paid the ultimate price for those efforts.

Uppermost in the queries this day of October 10, 03, in the Earth-bound players is, of course, our appearance in Zoronezh. That, of course, was several days prior, but has only come into your attention. Yes, we are the basketball players of the Cosmos and I have been telling you ones for months that we would begin to make Earth manifested appearances often and soon.

Ah, but mine ones are a bit offended; why in Russia and not in your village? Come now, you all know the answer to that question--because you ones shoot at us with missiles and interrogate and incinerate us when we show up on your lands. You ones still have much to learn about your placement. Bless and honor the ones who came before us for the payment has been most precious for their pioneering into your hostile places.

We are in your skys constantly--all over the map. We are totally accepted in every continent---even yours; 'tis only that you, the people, are not allowed to know. So be it. It is necessary to make our presence accepted elsewhere for your protection and from a place noted for closed information---still your news-casters take great sport and giggle and joke; you ones are in most serious trouble if you fail to "get with the program". There is nothing funny about nor prankster about our visits for the "A" Team is now coming in in full intent. You will recognize the truth of your Godness and honor the Laws of The Creation or your great numbers will perish. It will not be of our doing---YOU HAVE DONE IT UNTO YOUR OWN LIFE SOURCE.

Dharma, we must move right along on the document regarding your last great plague for our truth WILL be accepted; word WILL go forth and we will back it up as to resource so that no man can discount of it as invalid. Blessed are the ones who participate in this projection of truth unto his fellow man.

We note that in the descriptions of your news media, that the pictures utilized on your projectors are those of our beloved Eduard Meier, whom man has all but destroyed for the misadventure of trying to bring truth unto you. Well, dear ones, ye shall reap of that which ye sow. Too late smart, perhaps?

OUR NEXT BOOK, DHARMA, WILL BE CALLED AMERICA SLEPT HERE! SO BE IT AND SELAH.

I am going to have you write some things which will be most difficult for you, precious, for you are of us but you are so vulnerable to man's attacks. I can only request that those in the receiving of these documents use great caution with this scribe for the farther we push into truth, the more dangerous it is to her physical format. It is worse than we have pointed out in SPACE-GATE, ECONOMIC DISASTER, AND "SURVIVAL". YOU ARE SET UP TO HAVE KILLED OFF, AT LEAST A HALF TO TWO THIRDS OF YOUR POPULATION FROM AIDS--THE LAST GREAT PLAGUE. FURTHER, THE RUSSIANS HAVE THE KNOWLEDGE AND THE EQUIPMENT TO CURE THE DISEASE---DEVELOPED IT WITH YOU AND YOU HAVE THE SAME EQUIPMENT IN THE UNITED STATES TO INSURE NO DEATH TO ANY OF YOUR SO-CALLED LEADERSHIP OR FAMILIES THEREOF---ALL MEASURES WILL BE TAKEN TO SEE TO IT THAT YOU DO NOT HAVE ACCESS TO THE DEVICES UNTIL THE DASTARDLY DEEDS ARE DONE. FURTHER, YOU WILL NOT ONLY ALLOW THE GOVERNMENT TO SET YOU UP AND WIPE YOU OUT, BUT YOU WILL DEMAND THAT IT DO SO.

Your countries of Russia and the U.S. have been allies for some great long time now. Both caught in the trap of the other. You cannot, as a population, survive a nuclear war in which the Russians can annihilate you; and they are falling into the deadly economic trap that will finish them as a country; falling into the trap of the Top Secret Government of the U.S., the Trilateral Commission, The International Monetary Fund etc, etc, etc---(see all "Phoenix" Documents and Memoranda as mentioned above). Russia is now on its way to demise economically for all the low interest loans, grain and all those "exchanges" will have a very high price in the ending when they are owned by the "select" few. At which time there will be naught for them to lose and they will fight back. Further the Communist Chinese will enter the picture in great masses.

YOU ARE APPROACHING ARMAGEDDON, BROTHERS, AND YOU BETTER SEE OF IT FOR IT IS SOON TOO LATE TO DO ANYTHING TO MAKE YOUR JOURNEY MORE PLEASANT.

AIDS IS A MAN-MADE DISEASE! PERFECTED VERY CLOSE TO YOU DEAR UNSUSPECTING ONES AND IF IT IS NOT COUNTERED, IT WILL WIPE OUT HALF TO TWO THIRDS OF EARTH POPULATION---THE ONLY ONES WHO CAN COUNTER IT AT PRESENT ARE YOUR ENEMIES. FURTHER, THE LEADERSHIP IN ALL THE GREAT COUNTRIES WILL ALLOW A LARGE PORTION OF THEIR OWN POPULATION TO BE SNUFFED OUT----YOUR PLANET CANNOT SURVIVE WITH SUCH GREAT POPULATIONS AS YOU HAVE BRED. THE ANTI-CHRIST IS IN FULL SWING AND THE CHRIST FORCES CANNOT INTERFERE AT THIS POINT BUT WE

CAN ASSIST IF YOU WILL BUT ASK US AND ALLOW PARTICIPATION.

The evil ones do not wish to lose this planet, for it is the ideal playground; however, the planet, as you know it, will be emptied. The Earth Mother is in rebirthing into higher density and with her will go the awakened few. The ploy of the dark brotherhood is to lower the population in an effort to lessen the burden on the physical planet--hence the prophecies--WHICH, BY THE WAY, ARE IN THE VERY ACT OF BECOMING TRUE--LOOK CAREFULLY ALL ABOUT YOU AND READ THEM AGAIN!

AIDS is your last great plague! It is a man-made, genetically engineered virus that was both deliberately and accidentally introduced into the "selected" world population. It is not a venereal disease. It is not a homosexual disease. It did not originate from the African green monkey (it won't even grow in the green monkey). IT IS NOT PREVENTED IN CONTAGION BY YOUR CONDOMS AND IT WILL NEVER BE CURED BY VACCINE.

It is a blood carried, easily transmitted virus which mutates to suit every individual entity. It is sloughed off into the intestinal tract and thereby is the danger to the homosexual male. It is easily transmitted via saliva droplet and can live outside the body for at least two weeks and remain dormant almost indefinitely. It was introduced by your governments through great and wondrous smallpox inoculation programs in the world and into your U.S. homosexual population in '79 and early '80s by Hepatitis B programs in your gay communities. It is 100% infectious through hypodermic needle transference from infected to "clean". You do not have one or five AIDS viruses to deal with, you have at least 9,000 to the fourth power. Go ahead and demand "sterile" needles for your drug uses---"they" are just waiting for you to do that---you can get about 50 billion AIDS viruses on a pin head--it only takes one on the hypodermic needle and be assured, they will be on those sterile needles. The so-called "undesirable" population is fully intended to become extinct. Further, they will become so, for unless ones turn back unto truth and unto the Laws of God and The Creation in your actions and intent, we are not allowed to intervene. You will bring your moral behavior back under control and you will stop your degraded and base behavior life styles. Man does not have to have physical contact to LOVE another--be it man or woman; LOVE has naught to do with sexual foolish behavior. LOVE is protecting of any endangerment to another--the act of SEX behavior is self fulfilling lust and totally for pleasure of self. YE SHALL BE GIVEN TO REMEMBER SODOM AND GOMORRAH BEFORE THIS JOURNEY IS FINISHED----YE HAVE BEEN LED DOWN YOUR PROVERBIAL "PRIMROSE PATH" TO THE EDGE AND OVER THE CLIFF!

I make no judgment one way or another; I simply tell you how it is for we of these dimensions are given to know and have infinite data banks for backup.

Oberli, make sure that in the opening of this document, the credentials of myself and Commander Ashtar are given. We will be also in the pleasure of sharing with Sir Walter Russell and Sir Nikola Tesla--I will assume your readers already recognize of their stature. AIDS will never be brought under control except through light vibration of specific frequency attuned to each individual virus. It is most certainly not accepted medical technique and every effort will be made to stop successful completion of the mechanisms required. Funding will have to come from outside orthodox channels but there are ones who will dare.

Note that two of your California doctors received the Nobel Prize-----for work on genetic structure of cancer cells----thirteen years ago. DEAR BROTHERS, IN THIRTEEN YEARS FROM NOW, YOUR POPULATION WILL BE TOTALLY, IRREVERSIBLY DEVASTATED! THERE IS NO INTENT ON THE PART OF MEDICAL SCIENCE OR YOUR ORGANIZED GROUPS TO HAVE A CURE! THE CURE IS TOTAL SIMPLICITY AND WILL COST ALMOST NILL, YOUR MEDICAL COMMUNITY, YOUR DRUG COMMUNITY AND OTHER VARIOUS AGENCIES WILL BLOCK IT AT ALL COSTS. ILLNESS, CUTTING, BURNING AND NON-CURING IS YOUR WAY OF EXISTENCE AND THAT BASTION WILL NOT FALL SIMPLY TO SAVE LIVES.

I would, however, suggest the insurance companies look very carefully at funding this nonconformist method of treatment and cure for yes, it is going to work and if you don't work quickly the insurance companies of the world will be totally decimated. Then, add on those natural disasters which will be coming one upon another and you have the extinction of a business group.

"Hugo" will appear as nothing in comparison to that which is coming into thy realization within the next very short period of time. Climate changes of extremes, Earth changes and upheavals of mammoth proportions; winds, volcanos and earthquakes---all, one on top of another---and, you are in it NOW! It will just get more and more severe.

A good underground survival program can save your lives in the millions if you will get busy. If you shelter yourselves from atomic war, you can save yourselves from much of the earth-changes happenings.

Let us just suppose those in Carolina "Hugo's" path had had underground tunnel facilities as they have in Russia, China and Switzerland---they would now have complete rebuilding equipment, food, water, generated electricity and total security for everything that transpired on the surface. Before Hugo is forgotten you will have emotionally devastated populations in that area. Ones can handle the instant disaster but the overwhelming job and loss is too devastating to modern man who has dwelled solely in the luxury of an American existence. You cannot even survive without electricity any longer or heat yourselves without gas or power, ye have naught with which to pioneer in the midst of "everything".

These things can serve as warnings or they can just prove the point, whichever you ones wish to accept. You are in year three of your final countdown.

This document will be a most long and drearysome dissertation to most of you----most of your populace will not even read of it for that might interfere with your ball games or other important activities---well, soon you will have but one activity to attend--funerals! So be it!

We are knocking upon your door---it would behoove you to open it unto us and ask us in; call us "opportunity" and we have already been standing outside knocking for some fifty years---you are nearing the last of the petition to assist and if we turn from your door, ye cannot even comprehend thy plight.

All things brought forth from these dimensions can be checked and proven unto yourselves. It has been intentionally planned such. This scribe has no information, no names, no knowledge---we write the content and give unto you resources, whereby you can check these things out to your own truth and satisfaction upon your hard, cold desks and telephones. WE bring naught but truth, friends, and he who has ears to hear had best do so; and he who has eyes to see, had best use them for the time of hearing and seeing are at hand and you had better move up out of your fantasy dreamlands, little sleepyheads, for while you have been put into deep sleep thy world has crumbled about your ears.

WE FURTHER COME, TO DENOUNCE THOSE ONES WHO HAVE PERPETRATED UPON THE PUBLIC THE LIES OF OUR HOSTILITY. WE COME ONLY IN LOVE AND CARE FOR YOU, OUR FOOLISH LITTLE BROTHERS, WHO KNOW NOT TRUTH.

MAN WHO HAS GROWN IN ABILITY TO TRAVERSE THE UNIVERSE COMES NOT TO A TRANSITIONING PLANET SAVE BUT IN PEACE. THE STORIES OF HEINOUS ABDUCTIONS ARE FALSE STORIES TO BREED PANIC AND FEAR WITHIN THE POPULACE. NOT ONE PERSON HAS EVER BEEN LIFTED OFF YOUR PLACE EXCEPT IN GREAT LOVE AND PRIOR CONTRACTUAL AGREEMENT. STORIES TO THE CONTRARY HAVE BEEN TO FRIGHTEN YOU AND TERRIFY YOU OF OUR PRESENCE. THE ONES IN ZORONEZH WERE TERRIFIED; FURTHER, THE BOOKS OF HORROR SELL BETTER TO A POPULATION WHO NOW FEEDS ON SATANIC HORRORS AND HEINOUS VIOLENCE---MAN WILL CHANGE OR MAN WILL PERISH FROM THE FACE OF THIS EARTH!

SO BE IT AND SELAH. FOR AS THE PROPHECIES HAVE BEEN BROUGHT FORTH UNTO YOU ONES BY MANY, MANY ONES PRIOR TO MY CONTACT, THESE THINGS WILL COME TO PASS UPON YOUR PLACE IN THIS TIME FOR AS IT IS SO WRITTEN, SO SHALL IT COME TO PASS. WHAT YOU DO ABOUT IT IS OF NO CONSEQUENCE TO US, WE COME IN THE SERVICE OF THE CREATOR SOURCE AND IN BEHALF OF EARTH CREATION. THE CHOICE IS YOURS; CREATOR GRANTED YOU FREE-WILL CHOICE AS THY DIVINE GIFT---HAVE YOU USED IT WELL? MAN CAME AS CARETAKER UNTO THIS WONDROUS PLANET---HAVE YOU TENDED IT WELL? YOU ARE THE TEMPLE OF THE CREATOR; HAVE YOU HONORED THAT STATION? SO BE IT FOR IT IS IN THE FINISHING!

Go Dharma, that you might have a break and prepare for this day for thy next days will be filled to overflow. We shall have frequent breaks but we must move most quickly---man shall be given the truth, dear ones, what he does with it is not of thy business, each shall make of his own that which he will.

I move to stand-by. You shall be prepared, please, to receive from myself, Ashtar, Sananda, Nikola and Walter. Do not be concerned, for your frequencies are long since attuned to our transmitter/receiver range. We must be about our Father's work, chela, and so shall we be.

COMMANDER GYEORGOS CERES HATONN TO STAND-BY

HATONN CLEARING FREQUENCY PLEASE. SALU

OUT

CHAPTER 3

REC. #2, HATONN

TUESDAY, OCTOBER 10, 1989 1:21 P.M. YEAR 3, DAY 055

Hatonn present to begin communique. I shall be called away from time to time prior to completion of this document, therefore, please be prepared to receive Commander Ashtar, Dharma. We will effort at keeping the segments to no more than three hours in length and I request that you not become involved with other distracting projects during the days required to put this information to print.

This is the most important one item facing mankind this day. As serious as your other problems may seem, if no one is left to experience them, they become most insignificant. You are into your LAST GREAT PLAGUE---AIDS.

I shall be setting many misconceptions to right and also will likely readjust some thinking regarding the matter of who has done what and to whom it is done unto. You continue to be people of the lie with little recourse, and the lies become more and more lethal; well, truth may be your only recourse and therefore, we shall spare no feelings or words for the survival of your peoples depends upon what we do about this horrendous problem.

Most of the opening information and description of your plight is already known upon your place in one format or another, but for all readers' information, much must be in repetition. You must have background, status, projections, prognosis and integration with the "times".

WHAT IS AIDS AND WHAT ABOUT A PLAGUE?

AIDS is, by all definition, a "plague"! It will affect society in ways that you cannot now even imagine. There is no cure within your grasp as a people and no prospects of a vaccine--both of which will be thoroughly discussed as we move along. Even by scientific optimistic projections it is not even hoped for within the next fifteen to twenty years, at best. It is projected by Public Health experts that over 2.4 billions of people, half the world's population, will die from AIDS viruses and mutations of those viruses within that period of time. Not a pretty picture by any standard.

Economic devastation is impending for the medical health systems, insurance facilities and all related services within the next decade.

Now, some shocking information for most of you newly interested readers who feel safe and secure with your singular relationships and the comfort of a cosy condom. If things do not change radically and immediately, what you are really destined for is extinction.

AIDS is NOT prevented, nor hardly even impacted, by use of condoms. AIDS is NOT a venereal disease. AIDS is NOT a homosexual disease and AIDS did not come from any monkey bite in far off Africa. It came right out of a man organized laboratory by cross breeding cattle and sheep viruses--(it will not grow in the green African monkey).

The AIDS virus was specifically requested, produced, deployed, and now threatens extinction of the species. You are headed for the worst catastrophe in the history of your world. Yes, there is a cure---100% cure, but your government and controlling factions will not allow it to come forth---it is being held secretly for the privileged few. And since the purpose is to annihilate selected groupings of persons deemed unsuitable, you will not be given the methods of cure until it so pleases your guardian leaders.

As background for this material I must request that you obtain prior writings by myself and Commander Ashtar as well as some of the higher dimensional entities. If you don't know what the problem is, you cannot even hope to solve it. We are not in the book business but our intent has been to give information forth in proper sequence that you might understand our truth and as the material gets heavier and heavier we don't have to continually deal with disbelief in our status.

HOW DID IT GET HERE?

The first officially diagnosed case of AIDS was in San Francisco in 1981. Actually, it went something like this: The AIDS virus appeared in New York in 1978, San Francisco and Los Angeles in 1980. It appeared in young, white, male homosexuals who were between the ages of twenty and forty and permiscuous in behavior. Simultaneously with its appearance, there was conducted a Hepatitis B vaccine study in New York in 1978 and in San Francisco and Los Angeles in 1980---among young white male homosexuals who were between the ages of twenty and forty.

You must surely ask yourself if there is a relationship between the Hepatitis B vaccine study of the United States and the subsequent outbreak of AIDS in the same population groups and at exactly the same time.

Further, this followed right on the steps of the outbreak of the disease in third world areas such as Africa and Haiti in the 1970s. West coast gays, particularly from San Francisco, made Haiti a main playground and vacation spot during that ensuing period of time, thereby being hit from two directions.

WELL, HOW DID IT GET TO HAITI?

I am going to tell you and then I will explain about viruses and why you are in such devastating predicament.

In your mid 1970s the outbreak of smallpox in Africa was epidemic and spreading into many other sectors. An organization was created called the World Health Organization (WHO), which made an all out effort to inoculate thousands and thousands of people, among which were some 15,000 Haitians who were working in Africa at the time.

Now, before you jump off into accusations of "assumptions" let me point out a few things which are readily documented in hard physical fact and I expect you to do some checking for your own comfort and confirmation.

ABOUT THE SO-CALLED AIDS VIRUS/VIRUSES

You have to have some understanding of viruses, bacteria, human cell origin, tissue culture and manipulation of all those things within the laboratory. I hereby give confirmation to Dr. Robert Strecker for this simple and most adequate discussion regarding the subject. He has isolated the mechanism and actually knows, further, the cure in concept. We shall help in fleshing out that which is missing from the present data.

In the addressing what the AIDS virus is, the virus has a morphology which is actually a D-type retrovirus. So what are viruses? Some of you people are convinced, and I shall not confuse you, that viruses are the smallest replicating micro-organism. That means they are thought to be the smallest replicating organism that require other cells in which to grow themselves.

That viruses are not capable of reproducing themselves on their own, outside of living tissue, is the conviction of the scientists today. Viruses must inhabit another cell for potential growth and reproduction.

Bacteria, fungus, and some other organisms are actually capable of growing outside of tissue, in other words, they don't have to inhabit other tissue to reproduce themselves. They can grow on tissue culture plates such as bacteria. The viruses must grow inside of tissue which requires that there be living human or animal tissue in which they may replicate.

Retrovirus means that it is a small replicating organism which grows inside of living tissue. So what does the term "retro" mean? In the case of this particular virus, it stands for the fact that contained within the AIDS virus, and other so-called human retroviruses, or other animal retroviruses, are small enzymes known as reverse transcriptase. That is where the word "retro" comes from. The reverse transcriptase, which is where the "re" comes from "reverse" and the "tro" from transcriptase. That is an enzyme in the AIDS virus which actually is responsible for duplication of the genes of the AIDS virus which are in an RNA form, different from human form. Human genetic material grows in a DNA form.

If the AIDS virus is to insert itself into human material, somehow after infection of the cell, what happens is this enzyme duplicates the RNA of the AIDS virus into a DNA form and actually inserts that into the human DNA. The AIDS virus genes get in and are actually duplicated into DNA form, copied by the reverse transcriptase. That information is then inserted into the genetic makeup of the human cell. This is now an AIDS virus residing within the human genes which then sends out a signal for production of a NEW AIDS virus. Read carefully---NEW AIDS VIRUS!

Beyond AIDS the genetic information of all retroviruses is copied into the DNA form by the reverse transcriptase inserted into the genes and subsequent production of new viruses.

Let me generalize a bit of information here for better understanding. Virology is the study of viruses which deals with tiny living organisms visible only with the use of the most powerful electron microscopes on your planet as you now recognize the scientific limitations. Millions of AIDS viruses can easily fit onto the head of a small pin. The AIDS virus is particularly deadly to you humans because of its ability to not invade and neutralize human cells, but the virus' ability to put its own genetic material inside the human cell's genetic structure, thereby allowing the virus to use the human cell as a kind of virus factory, reproducing from a human cell's raw materials.

Unlike larger organisms, as with bacteria, viruses do not respond to conventional medical treatment. Much like your common "cold" virus, it cannot be treated effectively by drugs. The difference, however, in its attack is that the immune system is overwhelmed, which I will also present here.

Dharma, might we please have a break at this point and resume at a later session? Thank you.

SALU, HATONN TO STAND-BY PLEASE

CHAPTER 4

REC. #1, HATONN

WEDNESDAY, OCTOBER 11, 1989 7:00.A.M. YEAR 3, DAY 056

Hatonn present to continue. Let us press right along, please.

Do you think perhaps Mr. Donald Trump might feel, today, that he may have a higher purpose than building boats and plucking airlines? Will he credit where due or will he just be smug and think, "More good old Trump luck?" So be it.

Also, dear friends, KNOW that there is far more going on with the space shuttle launch, most certainly, than that which is on your news. I am not at liberty to inform you ones, there are ones in that sector who are aware and doing what they can. We are right on duty also, so they may be foolish enough to launch but the launch has been postponed until it can be more carefully considered. I'm sorry, Mr. Beardon, but we are your invisible light balls present at each launch. However, the Russians have the capability of tuning into the proper frequency and, as in the case of the Challenger explosion, knew it was going to blow and got out of the area to avoid blame. I shall speak of these things at length later in this document.

We will comment each day, or at least every few days, on what is REALLY going on in your news if that would interest you receivers.

I would say at this point that nobody needs sabotage your airships or technical equipment; your own equipment builders are quite effective at incompetent fabrication and repair. You live in one gigantic death trap of altered mind capacities. We stand by to retrieve life forms and disarm death weapons intended for space.

YOU WERE TOLD ON THE 19TH OF AUGUST, 1987, DHARMA, THAT FIRST WE WOULD BE DENIED AND THE COVER-UP CONTINUED AS LONG AS POSSIBLE, THEN WE WOULD BE RECOGNIZED BUT GROUNDWORK WOULD HAVE BEEN LAID TO TERRIFY THE POPULACE AND THEN, A MAMMOTH EFFORT WOULD BE MADE TO BLAME US FOR ALL YOUR `GREMLINS' IN THE WORKINGS, ALL CHEMICAL AND BIOLOGICAL WARFARE, FAMINE, ELEMENTAL DISRUPTIONS, ETC., ETC., ETC. THIS IS WHY WE ARE BRINGING FORTH THIS INFORMATION AND COUNTERING IT---IT IS WIDELY KNOWN THAT THEY WOULD BRING CHARGES AGAINST SPACE COMMAND FOR AIDS. THEREFORE YOUR LEADERS LEAVE US NO ALTERNATIVE OTHER THAN TO TELL YOU WHAT YOU FACE AND WHY YOU FACE IT.

Dear ones, it is truth which now comes to you in a daring book "OTHER LOSSES". In Germany, following the allied take-over, well over a million

German soldiers, most who knew nothing about camps or war, were tortured and kept without food or water until they slowly died in agony in U.S. Army prison camps. Oh, you don't want to know that? Did you want to know what really happened in Viet Nam? UNLESS YOU GOOD PEOPLE OPEN YOUR EYES AND MAKE SOME CHANGES, IT IS GOING TO GET WORSE AND WORSE AND WORSE.

Do you actually think the mess in drug infested Panama and Mr. Noriega is an accident?

Can you believe that even your "good" people are totally irresponsible? If you have read, as we have requested, "SURVIVAL IS ONLY TEN FEET FROM HELL" by Commander Antheose Xandeau Ashtar, then you will enjoy this note: Dr. Arthur Robinson, of "Robinson and North" who gave you a survival shelter blueprint in "FIGHTING CHANCE", went home to his dwelling location, gave out--free of charge--hundreds of books and offered to build, free of charge, a shelter system at the local school to house a hundred people. Not only did the community not build a shelter system, they wouldn't even allow his contribution to be built-----"WHO WOULD CHOOSE THE HUNDRED SURVIVORS?" ----!

DOES IT NOT MAKE YOU FEEL A BIT HELPLESS? OH, WOULD YOU EVEN BUILD THEM TO "PROTECT YOURSELF FROM THESE AWFUL INVADERS FROM THE COSMOS"! WE CARE NOT "WHY" YOU BUILD THEM, WE JUST WANT YOU TO BUILD THEM FOR YOU ARE THE CHOSEN ONES TO REBUILD AFTER THE BIG BANG COMES DOWN. WHAT DOES IT REQUIRE TO GET THE ATTENTION OF MAN? WELL, WE PLAN TO KEEP FURTHER MURDER OF OUR PRE-ENTRY CORP TO A MINIMUM--WE ARE NOW COMING FORTH IN HOLOGRAPHIC FORMAT SO WE CAN GET AWAY EQUALLY AS QUICKLY AS WE SHOW UP. NOW SEE IF YOUR BIG BOYS CAN FIGURE THAT ONE OUT!! WHEN WE MEET, ANY MORE, WITH YOUR LEADERS, WE DO NOT MANIFEST IN TOTAL FORMAT FOR WE DARE NOT GIVE YOU, ANY LONGER, EQUAL ADVANTAGE---YOUR ONES HAVE NO BASE OF FAIRNESS AND DO HAVE UNLIMITED ILL INTENT.

* * * * *

Let us now continue with our discourse regarding AIDS, and viruses in general.

Virology, of course, is the study of viruses. This deals with these tiny living organisms (which happen to be crystalline `crystals'). Millions of viruses can fit nicely on a pinhead -- (and dance with all those angels which also fit on a pinhead). It is most difficult to be a virologist because the treatment of virus disease falls outside your known medical capabilities.

The AIDS virus is particularly deadly because of its ability to NOT `invade and neutralize' human cells, but the virus' ability to put its own genetic material inside the human cell's genetic structure. Now with this reminder let us continue.

EFFECT ON HUMANS

Basically the immune system of humans is broken down into two parts. One is labeled B-cells, after the word which is its full label (you ones love dearly your alphabet), and the other is called T-cells. Let us just say that the B-cells control antibodies which control "B"acterial infections.

T-cell systems control the arisal of your opportunistic infections such as the pneumocystis carinii pneumonia and Kapose's sarcoma---diseases which ultimately kill the human entity. You can also lump tuberculosis in the grouping, but there are different methods of curing and controlling some of these other invaders than you have for the AIDS mutant viruses. As you recall, it was not always simple to treat tuberculosis, syphilis, etc.---it becomes more difficult today for you misuse your "miracle" drugs and propagate more sturdy and defiant strains of even those "curable" diseases.

Once the AIDS virus infects the human body it <u>selectively</u> destroys the T-4 cells. The T-4 cells are a mandatory portion of the human T-lymphocytic system. This is your system that assists you in the controlling of cancers, fungus invasions and others organisms. It is all too complex for Hatonn to detail herein for that information is readily available and this is written for alternate purposes.

The AIDS virus <u>selectively</u> destroys these T-cells. Now, briefly look at the incidence of these new, so-called, human retroviruses which plague you these days. I shall not do this alphabetical/numerical system as purely as would your scientist, but I will make of my point, I believe, and you ones do not ordinarily count with Roman numerals. First on the new assembly line is HTLV-1, which is responsible for T-cell leukemia. Then, HTLV-2 which is responsible for "hairy-cell" leukemia. Then, the big one, HTLV-3---which you label the AIDS virus.

Now, if you put HTLV-1 into a tissue culture it causes things "to grow and proliferate" and therefore you are likely to find T-cell leukemia.

If you place HTLV-2 into a tissue culture you will have a "hairy-cell" leukemia develop.

Now, the big one, HTLV-3. Woops, in a tissue culture this one is not proliferative--it is destructive. If placed in a tissue culture and checked a few days later the culture would be dead.

This is basically what happens in your human species because you are not much more than a walking tissue culture. Suppose you have a human who gets infected with the AIDS virus, the virus will kill off his T-4 lymphocyte cells, and in turn destroy the thymus gland in all probability, and will leave the body immune suppressed--compromised--and open for invasion of infections such as your deadly pneumocystis carinii pneumonia or arisal of cancer, most likely in this instance, Kapose's sarcoma. These two diseases are the "fingerprint, or `hallmark'" of AIDS viruses.

It is the overall picture, however, which is devastating to the human species. Suddenly, there is a contiguous explosion of diseases, not just AIDS, but other retroviruses---HTLV-1, HTLV-2, HTLV-3, HTLV-4 (a relatively newly recognized AIDS virus which is also known as HIV-2) and, HTLV-5. You also have one which Dr. Strecker refers to as 1LL (one-look alike). It is a good label for it is a deceitful mimic of another).

AFRICAN GREEN MONKEY VS. TRUTH

Here, I shall give Dr. Strecker further confirmation. (He doesn't need it, but I wish him to have it anyway.)

If you look at your planet's animal population and species, most particularly those immediately in your proximity, and evaluate and isolate the viruses which attack these animals you come up with your answer----AND YOUR PROOF THAT THIS AIDS DISEASE IS DELIBERATE AND MAN-MADE.

You will discover that in cattle there is a virus known as Bovine Leukemia Virus, which is exactly the same shape and identical in appearance to the HTLV-1 virus. It has an exact same dependence on magnesium as well as the exact same molecular weight. It has the ability to produce B-cell and T-cell leukemia in the bovine (cattle) population and is most proliferative in tissue cultures.

If you look at the bovine virus identical to HTLV-2 you will find another virus of cattle which has the same exact shape, the same magnesium dependency, the same basic appearance, the same molecular weight and produces "hairy-cell" leukemia in cattle.

Now, if you look further back, you will discover a virus known as Bovine "visna" virus, which has the exact same appearance as AIDS virus; the same molecular weight, morphology, magnesium dependency, etc. In 1974, either bovine leukemia virus or bovine visna virus was producing pneumocystis carinii pneumonia in one of your higher apes, the chimpanzee. (DO NOT CONFUSE WITH THE AFRICAN GREEN MONKEY.) But that, friends, is AIDS! You now have HTLV-4 which represents a recombination between visna and HTLV-2, or bovine syncytial virus, which is a new AIDS virus, and HTLV-5 virus and a mirror virus (look alike).

In simple terms, the AIDS virus attacks and destroys T-4 cells. Those are the cells within the body of living animals (humans included) that protect against the development of cancers, as such. In persons infected with the AIDS virus there is T-4 cell destruction and subsequent development of specific types of cancer---Kapose's sarcoma and pneumocystis carinii pneumonia, "the AIDS hallmarks"---which are always "lethal".

There are numerous other deadly retroviruses besides the actual AIDS virus, which are infecting humans and causing cancers, including cancer of the blood----leukemias. These human cancer causing retroviruses, including AIDS, are identical to animal viruses -- but not the African green monkey. They are from cattle and sheep, labeled as bovine and visna viruses. IF I WERE YOU ONES, I WOULD BE VERY NERVOUS ABOUT THIS TIME FOR YOU SHOULD BE MOST DISTURBED INDEED!

HOW DID ANIMAL VIRUSES GET INTO HUMANS?

Ah so---could there be foul play afoot? Cattle? Sheep? Where, then, goes the touted cause of AIDS, the African green monkey? Who would lie to you lovely, trusting citizens of the world "brotherhood" of man?

If you look at the genetic structure of the AIDS virus, the genes don't even look like a monkey's----they genetically appear *exactly* like bovine leukemia virus of cattle and/or visna virus of sheep.

These are retroviruses of animals and these viruses are known to cause "brain-rot" in sheep and leukemia in cattle. Therefore, if you cross these two viruses you produce AIDS virus. Only, your local AIDS expert will tell you otherwise and your politicians, physicians, pharmaceutical houses etc., etc.--will also vehemently disagree; but your veterinarians will agree!

If you have bovine leukemia virus on one hand and visna virus on the other, and you simultaneously infect a human tissue culture, what is produced is not only the original parent, bovine leukemia virus and visna virus, but every possible recombinant that will grow (and a lot that won't grow or reproduce which are called "incompetent"). An example is most simple in concept; you are each a recombination of your father and your mother and are *direct* descendents of those parents--50-50. These viruses "pair" to recombine and thus create a myriad of downstream offspring that are each slightly different---in other words, they are not "clones".

THIS WAS *PREDICTED*

A writing in Lancet, in 1956 by Mcfarland Burnett read as follows: "The human implications of what is going on in this sophisticated universe of tissue culture cells, bacteria and the viruses, are at best dubious; at most, frankly terrifying." (My ones, please recall I told you that in the 50's, in Israel, life had been created in a test tube! Hold this most dearly in your hearts; for if you can produce life you can ultimately produce death (of the soul essence) and you have now done that, also. THAT, FRIENDS, IS UNACCEPTABLE!)

Further, the author urged careful consideration about incorrect medical dogmas. In the case of AIDS you had best hold these assumptions in truth. Orthodox medicine in AIDS will annihilate your species.

Prediction? Just a bit more: "Regardless of your beliefs in the origin of man, being that of an evolutionist or a creationist, the author raises an alarming point about the manipulation of mankind through genetic engineering. Medicine must make use of all of the sciences, but it must also recognize the limitations that the process of evolution and the nature of man places on the utilization. It is a hard thing for an experimental scientist to accept, but it is becoming all too evident that there are dangers in knowing that which we should not know." So be it! One further comment from me; whether you are a "creationist" or an "evolutionist" you are not ready to accept the truth that it is NEITHER way---therefore, you must understand that you are just coming into knowledge---it would, therefore, be nice if at least a few of you could survive to move on into truth.

If you are a "creationist", how dare you think you can *improve* on God's work? If you are an "evolutionist", how dare you think you can produce an *instant fix*?

Oh yes, it was most explicitly *PREDICTED* that you would get yourselves into this mess---most explicitly. It was said by one of your doctor's at the end of an address on the subject: "We who are about to die, salute you." So be it! Will you move as easily into this slaughter trap as you have all the others to this point? If so, I neither salute nor condone your behavior. If you pitch in with some backbone and action I will stress, "We who are about to LIVE, salute you and `WELCOME ABOARD'!"

TO YOU WHO HAVE HONESTLY PETITIONED GOD FOR INPUT AND ANSWERS IN BEHALF OF YOUR FELLOW-MAN---HERE WE ARE, YOU HAVE IT DONE, BROTHERS, RECOGNIZE THE RESPONSE FROM CREATOR WHICH NOW COMES FORTH! SO BE IT AND SELAH. WE OF THE HIGHER COMMAND SALUTE YOU WHO RISK AND DARE!

A break, please, Dharma. I would like the prior statement to sink-in a bit before moving onward. Salu. Rattle my chain, chela, when you are prepared to continue. Hatonn to stand-by.

CHAPTER 5

REC. #2, HATONN

WEDNESDAY, OCTOBER 11, 1989 5:00 P.M. YEAR 3, DAY 056

Hatonn to resume.

A QUESTION OR TWO

First, I will respond to a question most often asked of me from Dharma's chair---why? Why are we doing this? We have exposed her to every secret intelligence agency, the government, the financial community, the Trilateral Commission, The International Monetary Fund, The Foreign Relations Council, told the secrets of the U.F.O. cover-up, gone against the government in survival fraud, told the truth about Immanuel, gotten every religious group ready to crucify her, cost her all her friends for they get frightened and drop away one after another, and now we shoot buckshot and flaming arrows at the Gods of the medical temples, as well as the government--what's left? Well, the legal system, but we will get there, also! We will probably also give you a blow by blow of "why this and that war", along with the biggest fraud of all----the war on drugs.

MY, HOW COMFORTING!

Dharma, they have killed you numerous times over the past several years---and you are still writing. I know that it is frightening, but you must also know that if you use caution and follow instructions, keep thy visitors most minimal---even thy true friends, and keep away from crowds and the major cities, we can tend you quite well. It does get more difficult, chela, but we must do that which must be done. You are directly attached to one or the other of us at all times, to Sananda at all times, to me at all times and now to which other is writing. If you are so much as touched, I am touched---more security than privacy, but ye are blessed for thy service. All of you in the service are likewise attended, you just are not given to remember the fulness of your contracts--it is far better that way. So be it.

Well, dear one, we will give you more than a firing squad--we also give you protection. It is, however, why everything must be released in snap, snap order--so that ones know you could not have written it. I have the load, little sparrow, you just keep the fingers moving.

GOVERNMENTS WILL BLAME ALIENS

* * * * * WE ARE GIVING YOU THE FACTS BECAUSE THIS IS A MAN-MADE, HEINOUS SHROUD OF PENDING DEATH YOUR OWN ONES HAVE PERPETRATED AGAINST MANKIND---AND THE INTENTION IS TO BLAME IT ALL ON SPACE ALIENS---COUNT YOUR DAYS; IT IS COMING VERY SOON WHEN THEY CAN NO LONGER RIDICULE OUR PRESENCE AWAY! * * * * * THERE ARE ONES IN THE PLANNING OF RELEASING IT FROM YOUR SPACE VEHICLES AND FURTHER, PLACING ONE OF YOUR OWN SPACE REPLICAS ABOVE ONE OR MORE OF YOUR CITIES IN ORDER TO MAKE YOU BELIEVE WE HOLD YOU HOSTAGE! * * * * * I WOULD MOST SURELY APPRECIATE ALL OF YOU IN THE READING OF THIS DOCUMENT SPREADING TRUTH INSTEAD! THANK YOU MOST HUMBLY!

What do you suppose they (the secret government) are going to tell you when all the captured ships come out of your secret hangers? You have our galactic craft in every major air base. You have killed our crews and the little ones from Reticulum came in such love and trust and walked into the waiting trap. You must hope they do not choose an eye for an eye! And how about those beauteous ones who transmute chlorophyll which you incinerated?. What about your own humans who knew too much and you killed and set up the parts to incriminate your space brothers? Pray, brothers, that God does not insist on the same type of reaping as in the sowing or your species won't make it comfortably through without paying a bit of karmic debt. Thank God on your bended knee that God, Sananda Immanuel, is the great judge for your leaders shall not get what they most surely deserve--and you? What about you? Who has elected those leaders and allowed the world to come into this state of disgrace and degradation? Who drinks the spirits to drunkenness, visits the prostitutes, have become the prostitutes in all manners of ways, killed thy brother if even by neglect, and who has taken the animal's life for your sport and blasted holes in your mother source for your greed and pleasure, who has acted in deceit, greed and thieved another's possessions and rightful substance? SO BE IT!

NAY, YE SHALL NOT TURN US AWAY BECAUSE OF THOSE WHO HAVE BETRAYED YOU. FOR WE SHALL NOT LEAVE OF OUR BROTHERS UPON YOUR PLACE TO BE FURTHER PERSECUTED OR MARTYRED. YOUR GOD WILL NO LONGER STAND SILENT, AND ONES WHO WOULD TOUCH OF OUR WORKERS AND SCRIPTORS HAD BEST STAND IN CAUTION, FOR IT WILL NOT BE LONGER TOLERATED. I, HATONN, AM OVER NINE AND A HALF FEET TALL AND TOTALLY BULLET-PROOF! TRY ME! I THINK THE SAYING IS, "MAKE MY DAY"! NO, DHARMA, OBERLI AND OUR OTHERS ON YOUR PLANE ARE NOT. HOWEVER, TANGLE WITH THEM AND YOU DIRECTLY TANGLE WITH ME! THAT IS, FURTHER, WHY YOU PROTECT THEIR POSITION FROM KNOWN ENEMIES.

WE APPRECIATE THE GOVERNMENT AGENCIES WHO KEEP THEM UNDER CONSTANT SURVEILLANCE FOR IT IS OBVIOUS WE HAVE NO INTENT OF OVERTHROW, ONLY INFORMATION IN A MOST PASSIVE MANNER--WE ARE NOT HOSTILE AND IF THEY SILENCE THIS ONE, THEY ONLY PICK UP ANOTHER MORE DANGEROUS TO THEM, FOR ALL INFORMATION IS ALREADY PUBLIC AND NOW THAT SO MANY OF YOU KNOW IT YOU CAN BRING IT FORTH WITH EVEN MORE ATROCIOUS EVIDENCE.

I HEREBY DEDICATE THIS VERY DOCUMENT TO TWO WHO GAVE IT ALL IN THIS CAUSE; TED STRECKER, WHO WAS MURDERED BY GUNSHOT AND REPRESENTATIVE DOUGLAS HUFF OF ILLINOIS, WHO WAS POISONED. THERE ARE OTHERS, BUT I CONTINUE TO HONOR DR. ROBERT STRECKER WHO CONTINUES HIS WORK IN SPITE OF KNOWING HE IS A MARKED TARGET---REMEMBER, HOWEVER, THEY RECKON WITH US HENCEFORTH.

Enough, Dharma, let us write at least a bit more about AIDS as that is our subject at hand.

* * * * *

ADAPT A VIRUS

The central issue of the AIDS subject is: How could you adapt a virus--an animal retrovirus, say a bovine visna virus--to grow in a human being?

The National Institute of Health would have you believe as other AIDS experts, that the virus simply jumps species---from African green monkeys into humans by biting them about the body somewhere--somehow, and then it exploded all over Africa, et cetera.

Woa, wait a minute. Do they not also tell you that YOU CANNOT TRANSFER THIS VIRUS BY BITING OR BY SALIVA? Well, have you another explanation of how the African green monkey might have functioned? They say THAT was a bite and, further, infected through the monkey's saliva! I tell you at this point---THE AIDS VIRUS WILL NOT GROW IN AFRICAN GREEN MONKEYS UNLESS "THEY" HAVE NOW DEVELOPED A STRAIN SPECIFICALLY FOR THE AFRICAN GREEN AND INTENTIONALLY INFECTED THE POOR CREATURES TO COVER THEIR ASSETS. THAT IS NOT LIKELY, THEY ARE RARELY THAT EFFICIENT NOR EFFORTING FOR SOMEHOW "THEY" ARE NEVER CALLED TO ANSWER FOR THE LIES.

Let us make you cringe a bit now. Was the AIDS virus really "requested"? You be the judge:

A quote from your World Health Organization, published in 1972, said the following: "An attempt should be made to ascertain whether viruses can, in fact, exert selective effects on the immune function. The possibility should be looked into that the immune response to the virus may, itself, be impaired. And if the effective viruses damage, more or less selectively, the cells responding to the viral antigens." Oh, well, you don't know what that gobble-de-goop means?

It means: "Make a virus that selectively inhibits the T-cell system of man". That, friends, is AIDS. It is not a coincidence that you now have a pandemic of a T-cell destroying virus, which was, in a sense, predicted and requested.

I am now going to share the story of the London Times for those who might not have heard it, though it is spread around quite freely these days, but was totally ignored at the time of the publishing of the article. The article also addresses the question of possible "request" for such a virus!

LONDON TIMES, MAY 11, 1987

On May 11, 1987, on the front page of the London Times,in an article entitled "SMALLPOX VACCINE TRIGGERED AIDS", Pierce Wright announced that the AIDS epidemic may have been caused by the World Health Organization (WHO) small pox inoculation in the third world countries. The conclusion is, of course, that it is truth. The story is like this: Somebody had been hired by the WHO to investigate whether or not the WHO vaccine programs, which were responsible for the eradication of smallpox in Africa, may have been a contributing factor to the spread of AIDS in Africa. Evidently a researcher, who has remained anonymous, who was afraid to reveal his name, was hired by the WHO to investigate that study. He did a study over a period of a couple of years, wrote a report, submitted it to the WHO, was paid for his service and sent on his way.

A year or so later this researcher walked into the London Times and threw the report on Mr. Wright's desk. Mr. Wright is the science writer of the London Times (a most respected and prestigious paper). The man said, "If you *really* want to know what is going on with AIDS in Africa, here is the answer!" Further, it has now even become more widely reported that the WHO suspected that its immunization program against smallpox might be connected to the AIDS outbreak. Well you might guess that WHO buried that report and promptly fired the consultant---a man of international reputation. The Times pointed out some startling correlations: "The smallpox vaccine theory would account for the position of the Central African states as the most afflicted countries, while Brazil became the most afflicted Latin American country, and how Haiti became the route for the spread of AIDS into the U.S.

"Brazil, the only South American country covered in the eradication campaign, has the highest incidence of AIDS in that region. The correlation is extremely strong." The London Times is not given to overexaggeration as are your American media.

Well, this story caused an uproar and front page stories popped forth in all the papers in Europe, Latin America and other parts of the free world. Did you read about it? So be it! Why do you suppose the American people are being denied critical information which is widely distributed throughout most of the world? Are you ready for some hard facts?

Would your own people do things like this? Oh yes, dear friends, and have.

LOOK AT "DELIBERATE"

In your 30's and 40's in your country, the U.S.A., in Alabama, there was a study undertaken by the U.S. Health Service which enlisted black men who were infected with syphilis. Those black men were serially followed over the ensuing years. The important part of this story is not that they were followed but that they were followed after the availability of penicillin which would cure syphilis. MOST WERE *SPECIFICALLY PREVENTED FROM HAVING PENICILLIN WHICH LED TO THE INFECTION OF THEIR WIVES AND THE DEVELOPMENT OF CONGENITALLY INFECTED SYPHILITIC BLACK CHILDREN.* That is documented in a book I urge all of you to obtain: BAD BLOOD, by James Jones.

Oh, you say, that was a long time ago and they were "just" blacks who had played around and probably deserved it? Read on!

Between 1959 and 1970 there were over three hundred biological experiments conducted on U.S. citizens, documented in another book I ask you to get for confirmation: A HIGHER FORM OF KILLING, by Harris and Paxman. This excellent, well documented book documents the biological warfare history of the U.S. and has put bunches of it into book form. To say that your government or other governments are not capable of doing these kinds of experiments, is to be most foolish with thy head buried in the sand-bucket---remember, you can die of suffocation in the sand-bucket.

You do not wish to believe your own country could conduct heinous acts of vindictive, pitiless cruelty? Did I not tell you this very morning that there is another book you should obtain: OTHER LOSSES? Your own U.S. soldiers, under General Dwight D. Eisenhower, slowly starved to death over a million Germans in your prisoner camps---deliberately and without conscience. MOST OF YOU WILL ALSO INITIALLY BELIEVE THAT AIDS COMES FROM SPACE BROTHERHOOD! YOU HAVE BEEN PEOPLE OF THE LIE FOR SO LONG THAT YOU CANNOT COMPREHEND TRUTH!

That is a long way away and also a long time ago? OK, let's get a little closer, especially to you ones on the West coast, let us say in or around San Francisco. How about a naval vessel, under the direction of the Department of Health, without telling anybody, sprayed serrations marcescences bacteria into San Francisco, infecting everybody. The researcher who conducted the study concluded that the average San Francisco resident inhaled at least five thousand of the bacteria during that project---this was to demonstrate that

San Francisco is subject to a biological warfare attack. Sleep well tonight for what you don't know will kill you sooner than you think!

HOW ABOUT ACCIDENTAL?

Well, no, it has not been accidental but for information let us see how smallpox vaccine is produced. A cow is placed in a narrow stall where it cannot lick and contaminate the belly area. The belly is shaved and scraped to sub dermal depth, smallpox vaccine is dripped onto the area and it is left to fester for a period of time, say a week or so after scabs form. The belly area is again scraped and the scrapings collected, it is dried and prepared and you have your next batch of smallpox vaccine.

Now, here is your possibility. Any virus contaminating the cow, such as we have mentioned prior to this, could be present; bovine visna virus, bovine leukemia virus, bovine syncytial virus, etc. (Remote possibility unless deliberately infected initially with the virus.) Woops, now another ouchie: In 1981, it was announced that there had been a known contaminant of fetal calf serum by something called bovine visna virus. That means, friends, that at the same time AIDS was breaking forth, you had been having contamination of fetal calf serum with bovine visna virus. That further means that this virus was present not only in cows, but was present in the growth medium that was being used for tissue cultures worldwide. It means that fetal calf serum, which is like the growth hormone for human and other animal tissue cultures, was contaminated with a virus which is known to have direct identicology to AIDS.

Just a tad more mixing and voila, you have the jackpot!

LETS TALK NUMBERS

Retroviruses are unfamiliar to the medical profession, by and large, for they are most prevalent in animals. You will now find veterinarians heading up the AIDS research groups and a lot of disheartening information is flowing forth.

When you see an index case of Aids, it is a pretty good rule of thumb that there are ninety nine subclinical cases coming on and supporting that one on top, so to speak.

Let us say you have 50,000 cases of AIDS in the U.S. at a given time; that means you have approximately five million coming. What else can you know from that general rule in retrovirology? You know that the viruses which support that one index case on the top, say a ratio of 1 to 100, will work over an extended period of time, on the rule of thumb average, 20% of the life span of the species. For you ones, that is around 20% of some 70 years, which would be about 14 years or so. Data shows that that calculation is close.

IMPLICATIONS OF TIMING

It most certainly has major implications regarding vaccine development. You have to wait an extended period of time, some 14 to 20 years, before you can find whether or not the vaccine is working. You would have to wait 14 to 20 years before you could know whether or not your vaccine would let you die or save your neck. These are called "*slow*" viral diseases of humans and represent a major new kind of problem with which most medical doctors have little or no experience.

Year before last you had about 40,000 *DOCUMENTED* cases of AIDS. Last year 80,000 reported. So it appeared the doubling time was about once per year. Sorry, dear ones, it is more like every six months.

The statistics reported by your WHO in Africa are staggering. As a continent, Africa, through the "AIDS belt" and other areas, there are between 40 to 75 MILLION infected. If that doubles just every year, it means that within a couple of years the entire continent of Africa may well be infected and in 4 to 8 years, the entire continent of Africa could be expected to actually expire.

BACK TO THE POOR GREEN MONKEY

You still want to believe it came from the green monkey? Sorry, it could not have come that route. If some jungle monkey bit someone you would have to have a spread from the jungle into the cities---sorry, it is spreading from the cities into the jungle. You would have to know a secret; the ones most closely associated with those green monkeys are the pygmies. Funny, up until a year or so ago, the pygmies were almost clear of AIDS virus infection. THEY ONLY BECAME INFECTED AFTER CLOSE ASSOCIATION AND CONTAMINATIONS FROM PROSTITUTES FROM THE CITIES OR BY NEEDLE CONTAMINATION FROM INTRAVENOUS DRUG ABUSE AS IT SPREAD OUTWARD FROM THE CITIES.

Further evidence against the virus coming from the monkeys is found in the codon choices of the AIDS virus. That means that the genetic information of the AIDS virus, known as codon choices, are not found in monkeys. They are not found in monkeys and they are not found in man--they actually exist in visna virus and a few other viruses of a laboratory. That is why the genetic structure of the genetic material, the so-called information of the genes of the AIDS virus look like visna virus, as we already know, in bovine leukemia virus. All of these facts show that no monkeys did it---just some humans monkeying around a bit, I would say.

Dharma, enough for tonight. We will swing into "sex and drugs" on the morrow. I most surely wish every sexually active human could have this document before bedtime tonight---but we will do the best we can. You literally take your very life to the game room with you. Perhaps someday you ones may even learn to use "sex" for what it really is for and stop calling it Love. So be it and good evening.

Rest well for we shall please begin early as this is a long document and a most timely matter.

Hatonn to stand-by

CHAPTER 6

REC. #1, HATONN

THURSDAY, OCTOBER 12, 1989 7:30 A.M. YEAR 3, DAY 057

Hatonn present and ready to continue. I have need to remind you of a few points and also caution you.

SEPARATE FACT FROM VISIONARY

As ones come into your space, you must remain apart, Dharma, to some extent. We come to this place and to you, at this time, with facts regarding all of mankind and the horrendous changes coming about on your planet. We are contradicting, almost without exception, that which is standard false portrayal of information in numerous facets of life experience. IT WILL NOT BE CONFUSED WITH ANY SECULAR GROUPS, METAPHYSICAL CABALS, POLITICAL OR GROUP "MOVEMENTS". WE COME FORTH TO PRESENT TRUTH AND ACT AS A BROTHERHOOD OF PEOPLE. WE MUST HAVE NO ATTENTION SEEKERS OR SELF-PROCLAIMED DO-GOODERS PLACING YOUR AUTHORS INTO SELECTED "CAMPS". WE ARE COME FORTH TO "ALL" WHO WILL RECEIVE OF THE MASTERS AND OUR COSMIC BROTHERHOOD; NOT TO SANCTION ANY GROUPINGS ON YOUR PLACE OTHER THAN TO COMMEND ANY AND ALL WHO FOLLOW THE LAWS OF CREATION AND THE LAWS OF GOD. SO BE IT!

This is why you, Dharma, will bear no cloak of a Hatonn, Ashtar, St. Germain, Sananda, Gabriel, Michael, et cetera---for you will experience all in truth and select and singular groups will move you toward dissension and conflict. Ones do not need even believe in my truth to recognize the truth of the messages and be most remarkable contributors--belief comes with unlimited acceptance and truth in knowledge--not singled out groupings of suspected cults and mystics.

The study of astrology is distorted and, let me remind you--you cannot trust star locations at the present time for most of your so-called major heavenly bodies are naught but our craft projected between them and you. This is not a time of dreamy eyed crystal gazers, mystics, soothsayers, fortune tellers and false gurus. THERE IS ONE GOD AND A WORLD IN HEINOUS TROUBLE, MOVING INTO TRANSITION. NO MORE AND NO LESS. WHAT YOU CHOOSE TO EAT WILL EFFECT YOUR BODY PHYSICAL AND THEREBY LIES THE WHOLE OF IT. THE DESIRE IS TO LIVE IN BALANCE AND HARMONY WITH THE CREATION---YOUR SOUL ESSENCE (INFINITE ENERGY BEING) IS COMPLETELY DIFFERENT IN NATURE OF EXISTENCE AND YOUR EATING HABITS, FOR INSTANCE, ARE OF NO CONCERN TO

US. FURTHER, ALL PHYSICAL FUNCTIONS ARE COMPLETELY CONTROLLED BY THAT CENTRAL ELECTRICAL SYSTEM CALLED MIND. AS IN AIDS, IT IS SIMPLE LIGHT FREQUENCY CONTROL OF GENETIC ENGINEERING AND STRUCTURING. THE MIND CAN CREATE AND THE MIND CAN DESTROY---OR, THE MIND CAN ENGINEER THE EQUIPMENT IN PHYSICAL FORMAT TO UTILIZE SEPARATE AND APART FROM INDIVIDUAL FOCUS. DO NOT PLACE VOO-DOO HOCUS POCUS ON ANYTHING--GOD IS INFINITE AND YOU, AS MAN, ARE HIS DIRECT FRAGMENTS. THERE IS NOTHING YOU CAN DO ON THE PHYSICAL PLANE THAT "BUYS" YOUR WAY TO THE HEAVENLY REALMS--ALL IS THROUGH THE GRACE OF "ALLOWING" FROM YOUR CREATION. WHAT YOU DO IN THE PHYSICAL ONLY ALLOWS THE KNOWING OF THAT WHICH IS REFLECTED IN THE HEART AND IT IS MOST CAREFULLY WATCHED.

YOU CAN EAT NAUGHT BUT WHEAT GRASS AND CHLORELLA, LOCUSTS AND HONEY FOR ALL YOUR DAYS, AND CARELESSLY HOP INTO BED FOR A LITTLE FUN AND GAMES FOR PHYSICAL PLEASURE AND NEGATE ALL THE GOOD INTENT OF THE DIET. YOU ARE ALSO VERY APT TO END UP WITH AIDS AND THEN BLAME GOD FOR YOUR MISFORTUNE. AIDS IS A "CONTACT SPORT", NOT A SEXUAL DISEASE----A *CONTACT* DISEASE AS EASILY SPREAD, OR MORE SO, THAN THE ORDINARY, COMMON THING YOU CALL "COLD".

I sorrow beyond words at that which your teachers are giving unto your babes---sex training at kindergarten and it's all alright if you just use a condom; further, if you become with child--simply choose to murder it on a clinical table. THERE IS NO TALK OF LOVING (LOVE IN TRUTH) RELATIONSHIPS, NO SUGGESTION OF SIMPLY MOVING INTO THE LAWS OF GOD AND CREATION AND USING DISCIPLINE AND SELF CONTROL---JUST SLIP ON A BIT OF FAKE RUBBER AND ALL IS WELL FOR YOUR LITTLE CHILDREN. OH YOU OF INSANITY--YOUR BABES ARE BEING MURDERED BY THIS INSANITY AND YOU IN THE LEAD. IT IS NOT ALRIGHT--FURTHER, EVERY FORM OF "LOVEMAKING" EXPERIENCED IN YOUR PLANE IS EVEN WORSE FOR INFECTION THAN SIMPLE MAN-WOMAN INTERCOURSE. IT IS CAPABLE OF ANNIHILATING YOUR SPECIES. YE ONES ARE REAPING THAT HARVEST WHICH YOU HAVE ALREADY PLANTED AND NURTURED AND YOUR PLANET CANNOT ENDURE THE POPULATION BURDEN--WE OF THESE REALMS HAVE GREAT COMPASSION FOR YOU LITTLE BROTHERS FOR YOU HAVE LOST YOUR WAY AND FOLLOWED YOUR DEADLY ENEMY.

Yes, Dharma, we are now visible all over your places. Each one of you can look into the heavens and see us in your night sky. We will be strategically stationed for easy viewing of multi light rotation and there will be ever increasing motion which you have previously discarded as "shooting stars". If there is a trail of particulate matter which glows as a comet, the craft is within your atmosphere. If the light is instant, exceptionally fast and leaves no substantial trail other than light movement, the craft is without your dense atmosphere----ENJOY! You certainly do not need rush off to Russia or Oklahoma--walk outside and simply peer to the heavens. Blessing upon you little ones coming into truth--the journey is most shocking indeed. So be it -- Au Da Pai Da Cum. There are millions of us out here waiting your petition, communication will become most regular and open as we move forward in attention. Those who "channel" in selected self aggrandizement for outrageous fees and attention shall surely fall by the wayside so ones of ours must look within at intent for the truth is for all--ALL! THE WORD MUST GO FORTH IN TRUTH *TO ALL MEN OF EARTH* NOT JUST A SELECTED FEW WHO CAN AFFORD THE PRESENCE OF AN ENTITY.

Let us please move back into our subject of the last great plague for it shall take a third to a half of the population of Earth in a very short span of "time" as you recognize "time", for much must be brought forth to stem the explosion.

* * * * *

CANCER

What is cancer? Well, let me assure you that Kapose's sarcoma and leukemia are cancers and they are the hallmarks of AIDS. Therefore, CANCER IS ALREADY A CONTAGIOUS DISEASE, TRANSFERABLE FROM ONE PERSON TO ANOTHER.

IF YOU BELIEVE YOU ARE SAFE BECAUSE YOU ARE NOT GAY OR PROMISCUOUS, OR BECAUSE YOU ARE NOT SEXUALLY ACTIVE, THEN YOU MISLEAD YOURSELF AND HAVE BOUGHT THE LIE!

Your scientists do not even know whether the transferral from one person to another is as a "free viral particle" or "a viral particle *inside* of a cell". That statement should terrify you. That is, in scientific ignorance, as profound as having a house building contractor not knowing whether a house is built or still in sticks and stones in a factory. There is a most spectacular difference. Therefore, when you get down to actually how this virus is being transferred, there is very little data or absolute knowledge.

They tell you that it is just a sexually transmitted disease, but they don't tell you anything about HOW the virus is getting across the membranes of either the man or the woman. Depending upon HOW it is getting across has a great deal to do with how really dangerous it is in the long run.

Well, I can assure you that you are so far from a cure of the disease by orthodox methods that it matters little in the long run. It will have to have a cure resource that is specific to ALL the mutations of the virus and specifically destroyed wherever they are located. Oh yes, there is a way to do that but all measures are being taken on earth level to prevent you from having it. There are some substances soon to be released in medication format which will give some assistance in maintenance and selective remission of active symptoms. I will discuss it in greater measure a bit farther on in this document when I get to the discussion of "combat and cure".

CONDOMS

Your greatest advocate of condom use in prevention of AIDS spread (and remember AIDS first exploded in the homosexual community) and control thereof, Surgeon General C. Everett Koop, made the following statements, "Prophylactics have extraordinarily high failure rates among homosexuals and offer them no assurance of safe sex." Later, he continued: "I don't like to acknowledge mistakes, and I don't want to use the word `mistake' in reference to that report - - but - - - -!" and then he further said, "Since the initial report was written, I am surprised to find a near complete lack of research on condom failure rates and causes. Only one study in progress has ever been designed to study the various issues of condom breakage (leakage and flaws) rates as they relate to AIDS."

* MOST COMMON MISCONCEPTION ABOUT AIDS VIRUS AND CONDOMS *

The most common misconception being foisted upon you people right now concerns sexually active people. You are told that if a man uses a condom the transference of the deadly virus is virtually eliminated. NOTHING COULD BE FURTHER FROM THE TRUTH. OF THE BODY FLUIDS THAT THE AIDS VIRUS IS FOUND IN, SEMEN CONTAINS THE LEAST! As fact, there is no significant amount of virus in anyone's ejaculate; perhaps about one virus per milliliter (a small portion indeed), a statistically irrelevant amount. A most copious ejaculation might produce only one or two viruses. Oh yes, you can substantiate in your own medical literature.

Now for worse news: You will here pretend that there are millions and billions of AIDS viruses in an ejaculation---woe is you; a condom is riddled with microscopic or larger holes natural in manufacture. THE *SMALLEST* HOLE FOUND IN CONDOMS ARE *TWO TO TEN TIMES LARGER THAN THE AIDS VIRUS !* IT BECOMES SOMETHING LIKE SHOOTING PING PONG BALLS THROUGH A BASKETBALL HOOP. *CONDOMS HAVE NOT, WILL NOT, AND CANNOT PREVENT AIDS*!

ASIAN TIGER MOSQUITO

Swamp fever, malaria, sleeping sickness - - - - all are borne by insects, namely the blood sucking mosquito. How is it that your "experts" tell you a mosquito does not carry AIDS?

The "father" of AIDS virus, bovine leukemia virus, and visna virus (sheep brain-rot virus) which is the "mother" of AIDS viruses, are borne animal to animal through blood-sucking vectors such as mosquitos.

The AIDS virus is most certainly spread through blood transferral by mosquitos and most especially the one known as Asian Tiger Mosquito, which in fact, was intentionally introduced into America specifically to spread the disease. It is most selective in its dinner plate and feeds mostly on human blood.

HOW ABOUT JUST MAKING A VACCINE?

How about a rundown on why there can't be a vaccine. The AIDS virus arose by recombination (mixing), of bovine leukemia virus and visna virus. The fact is that the genes of the AIDS virus contain approximately 9,000 base pairs, each base pair then has four choices, which means that there are 9,000 X 9,000 X 9,000 X 9,000 different AIDS viruses.

That means that instead of being a single virus, there is an entire "field" affect of viruses. There is a menagerie of viruses and that, of course, explains why every AIDS virus that has been isolated to date, is different.

Because they are all different therein lies the inability to isolate and produce a vaccine. AIDS is not a stable virus such as found in smallpox. Smallpox virus is the same today as a thousand years ago; same with chicken pox, mumps and measles and so forth. But the actual fact is that every AIDS virus isolated from *every* patient, more or less, has been different. The reason is because the virus reacts individually with the tissue within which it is growing. If it is growing within YOU it reacts and individualizes to fit YOU. They spontaneously mutate incredibly. There simply can be no SPECIFIC vaccine for there would have to be greater than 9,000 to the 4th at minimum. The recombinant nature of the beast precludes successful vaccine.

Further, the virus was created to have these characteristics. The virus was developed that would intentionally and collectively destroy the cells which are responsible for processing the virus and that is what AIDS is.

In your blood system you have cells which are called macrophages. It is the job of the macrophages to process this virus and present it to the T-lymphocyte for development of immunity. But what happens is that the macrophage cannot kill the virus, it grows inside the macrophage instead, the macrophage is then actually injecting it into other cells throughout the body. This leads to the death of T-4 lymphocytes as well as other cells, such as a rather important group of cells called the brain.

The defect is not primarily in the human lymphocytic system but rather lies in the macrophage system, the very cell responsible for processing the virus. The macrophage system's job is to process the virus and send it out in a form that the body can utilize to develop immunity. What is happening now is that if one is infected with AIDS virus and you have an antibody directed against that virus, those form a conjugate (reproduction) if you use a vaccination against the virus---that is the actual purpose of a vaccine, to produce these antibodies directed against the AIDS virus.

If you are vaccinated against AIDS, you have these conjugates formed, that allows the macrophage to ingest those antibody antigens *more easily.* The entire complex is ingested instead of the macrophage. The macrophage then processes the antibody, the virus grows inside the cell, and you die more quickly than if you had not been vaccinated. Vaccination against AIDS would be impossible for you at this time and would prove to be most detrimental.

You now have been given rational and clear reasons why an AIDS vaccine can never be practical nor actually developed. Firstly, you have astronomical numbers of mutations of the virus which means a specific vaccine, for a specific virus, cannot be made. Secondly, the way in which the virus is processed within the human body would make AIDS infection even more rapidly fatal when treated with a vaccine.

Of course this is disappointing to those efforting around the clock to make a vaccine. IS IT NOT MORE FOOLISH, HOWEVER, TO BLINDLY PURSUE A VACCINE CURE THAT CANNOT WORK, THEREBY DELAYING RESEARCH OF ALTERNATIVE METHODS OF TREATMENT AND CURE? FURTHER TAMPERING WITH THE VACCINE WILL ALSO CAUSE EXACERBATION OF THE DISEASE PROCESS ITSELF.

Dharma, might we have a break, please. This is a most unpleasant subject and we will perform better with regular pauses for whole body exercise and mental refreshment.

Hatonn to stand-by

CHAPTER 7

REC. #2, HATONN

THURSDAY, OCTOBER 12, 1989 4:45 P.M. YEAR 3, DAY 057

Hatonn responding, thank you. Now, to continue.

Here are some rather sobering facts for your Americans, alone. Over 30,000 Americans have already perished because they didn't know the truth about AIDS. Between seven and eight million Americans are already infected. One in 60 babies born in New York City is infected; one in 300 college students in America is infected; one in 20 aliens (and I don't mean extraterrestrial aliens) who are applying for amnesty in your country is infected, including the full sex spectrum---men, women and children. YOU ARE NOT GOING TO HEAR THESE FACTS FROM YOUR MEDIA, MY FRIENDS.

GO TELL IT ON THE MOUNTAIN!

The first place all of this information was taken, upon compilation, was to the medical and legal communities. Most were not even interested and certainly no one was prepared to risk their professional standing by making waves within the establishment. (WHAT IN CREATOR'S NAME IS THE MATTER WITH YOU PEOPLE?)

The material was then delivered to every Governor of every state, the U.S. President, the Vice-President (who is now President and still won't look for he has other fish to fry), the FBI, the CIA, the NSA, and selected members of Congress. The authors of the compiled material were swamped and bombarded with a total of three (3) replies from three governors; nothing from the government.

These brave men have been ridiculed at every turn. One informed the government that virtually every person testing positive for AIDS would die prematurely and painfully. The government said that was total nonsense. Government figures showed that perhaps ten percent at most would die from the disease. This was 1985.

In 1986, the government said that maybe 50 percent of those infected would die, in 1987 they said maybe 75 percent, and finally, in 1988 they agreed that AIDS IS VIRTUALLY 100 PERCENT FATAL! FEELING REALLY COMFORTABLE AND COSY?

This information was submitted time after time after time to the medical journals---all were refused for print. Even in Europe it was no better accepted even with the good old London Times on the correct side. Does anyone reading this remember a scorned physician who said, "DOCTORS,

WASH YOUR HANDS! YOU ARE INFECTING YOUR PATIENTS!" SO MUCH TOO LATE--SMART!

Getting your hands on this information from your life plane is a feat in itself because all efforts are made to hide it, bury it and destroy it--to the point of murder, and I jest not.

TV and radio stations refuse to allow mention or advertising of the material which I am giving you in this document. No price is large enough to bribe them to handle it. A national radio network did an interview with a famous talk show host and then the station refused to air it. Virtually every big name network television magazine show and all the syndicated TV interviewers and talk show hosts have said NO. Big city newspapers will not take any print ads telling about it and now you see what a mess you are in! Who do you think has squashed this material of truth? IT DOES TELL YOU THAT WE BRING YOU TRUTH, HOWEVER, DOES IT NOT?

WHY IS EVERYONE AFRAID? IT IS ONLY YOUR SPECIES HEADED FOR DEATH!

The excuse, of course, is that it is too controversial. IT IS TOO CONTROVERSIAL!?! "THEY" SAY THAT THIS INFORMATION, IF WIDELY DISSEMINATED, WILL CAUSE THE PUBLIC TO PANIC. **I WOULD MOST SURELY HOPE SO!**

If someone poisoned your national water supply and you and your family are on a direct course to death, all of your family, wouldn't you wish to know about it? Would you panic? Or, perhaps, you would more likely be outraged into action and find the ones who did it, do all you can to clear out the poison while taking all precautions in the interim--and then make sure it doesn't happen again.

THE ONLY ONES WHO ARE GOING TO PANIC IN THE WAKE OF THIS PUBLIC INFORMATION ARE THOSE SCIENTISTS WHO WILLINGLY OR OTHERWISE CREATED AIDS AND ARE NOW PROMOTING MISINFORMATION BY COVERING IT UP. IF YOU HAD CREATED (MADE) AIDS WOULD YOU TELL ANYONE? HOW ABOUT YOUR "SECRET" GOVERNMENT AND THE "SECRET" TRAITOROUS CONTROLLERS OF YOUR ECONOMY AND YOUR VERY LIFE ITSELF? IF YOU HAVE READ OUR PREVIOUS DOCUMENTS (LET US REFER TO THEM AS THE PHOENIX MATERIAL) THIS WILL COME AS ABSOLUTELY NO SURPRISE. DOES IT NOT TELL YOU SOMETHING IMPORTANT THAT WE OF THE COSMOS MUST TAKE THIS HIDDEN INFORMATION IN HAND AND PUT IT BEFORE YOU BLIND CITIZENS? HONOR THESE BRAVE ONES WHO DARE TO SAVE YOUR SPECIES FOR YOU ARE ON THE VERY BRINK OF ANNIHILATION. ONLY THOSE WHO CONTROL YOU AND ARE YOUR GREATEST INDIVIDUAL ENEMY, HAVE THE MEANS FOR SURVIVAL AND IT HAS BEEN COM-

PLETELY PLANNED WITH INTENTION OF DOING JUST WHAT IS BEING DONE UNTO YOU.

ENVISION YOUR LOVED ONES *DEAD*

Does the term "species annihilation" concern you? Well, you have the manner of doing exactly that in several ways, AIDS is but one but that is the one with which we are dealing at this writing so we will remain on that subject.

You must realize the implications, and realize that, unlike any other kind of disease ever known to man, past or present, AIDS can, if unchecked, KILL EVERY HUMAN ON EARTH. IT WON'T FOR THERE IS A WAY TO CURE IT AND IT IS KEPT FROM YOU. IT WILL ONLY KILL A THIRD TO A HALF OF THE EARTH'S POPULATION JUST AS YOUR "BIG BROTHERS" PLAN. DO NOT BLAME SPACE ALIENS---THESE ARE YOUR OWN SO-CALLED LEADERS!

Whether or not you like it or want to believe it or do not--whether you panic or quietly go to your coffin, and despite all precautions (for they give you the wrong information), the time will come when you WILL TEST POSITIVE FOR AIDS, and it will happen much quicker than you realize.

IT IS ALL AROUND OUT THERE

The number of AIDS-infected persons is doubling in far less than annually--in some areas, in only six short months. With seven to eight million Americans carrying the virus, you don't have to be a learned scientist to see how long you have there in the U.S.A.

Conservatively counting, Africa has approximately 100 million infected which are documented, another 50 - 75 million undocumented.

Brazil as a country is in very serious jeopardy because during the 1970s all the transfusion blood supply was shipped in from Africa. Further, the WHO conducted a large scale smallpox vaccination program there in the 1970s.

Southern Japan has over 30% infected but because of financial implications it is kept well hidden from the media.

Russia is now reporting AIDS as a problem and no one can enter Russia without a current negative blood test for AIDS.

Cuba has set up concentration camps for the AIDS-infected and they are already overcrowded.

Haiti, of course, is ravaged by AIDS; more than 15 percent of the total population is infected and worsening daily.

A leading "Guru" in India is advocating *death* by separation and starvation to any infected person.

Every nation on earth (excepting perhaps Iran, who wouldn't report it if they had 100% infection rate), is reporting a growing problem and is desperate for help. It is on every continent, every sub-continent and every island chain---Pacific and Atlantic.

NOW WHY DO YOU SUPPOSE THE MEDIA OR GOVERNMENT WON'T TELL YOU THESE THINGS? COULD THERE BE SOMETHING QUITE "FISHY" AFLOAT? WILL YOU PANIC AS THEY SUPPOSE YOU WILL OR WILL YOU STAND UP AND GET BEHIND THE CURE FOR THIS THING?

IS THERE HOPE?

Of course there is hope---not for a third to a half of the population for everyone has waited too long to act but of course there is--it already is in existence and set up and operating for the very select few and yes, the brave researchers who have given every waking hour, every cent they can beg or borrow are within a breath of having equipment in completion---WE WILL HELP THEM WITH INFORMATION TO ASSIST IN THE AREAS WHERE THEY ARE LACKING. YOU COULD SAVE MILLIONS AND MILLIONS BUT PROBABILITIES INDICATE THAT YOU WILL NOT RESPOND QUICKLY ENOUGH FROM YOUR NAP OR BALL GAME.

If you are waiting for your government to create a "magic bullet" you may as well toss in the hope along with the crying towel.

Let me briefly refresh your memory on some serious difficulties. AIDS viruses are "recombinant retroviruses". Very simply, that means they have the ability to recombine with the genes of any cell they enter and the offspring or new viruses they form are different from the parent viruses. HTLV-3 alone (that is the most common American AIDS virus) has the mathematical ability to change itself 9,000 X 9,000 X 9,000 X 9,000 times (9,000 to the fourth power). THE COMMON COLD RECOMBINES MUCH LESS FREQUENTLY AND YOU DON'T HAVE ANYWHERE NEAR A CURE FOR IT AFTER OVER A HUNDRED YEARS OF EFFORT.

FURTHER, DOES IT MAKE SENSE TO ENTRUST THE CURE FOR AIDS TO THE SAME PEOPLE THAT CREATED IT? AND HOW MANY FOXES DO YOU LOCK UP IN THE HENHOUSE EACH NIGHT?

Hope? Yes, more than that there is a quick, simple and relatively "free of cost" cure. It is an alternative, non-allopathic, non-drug modality based on Raman spectroscopy. In fact many experiments are going on currently and show great promise. Unfortunately, your government takes a dim view of any type of treatment for any type of disease, let alone AIDS, that does not conform to its rigid rules for acceptance, registration, and legalization---not to mention a corner for the giant pharmaceutical houses. Well, they might reconsider an allopathic treatment if it is presented by a sanctioned drug company or university. Friends, it simply is not going to happen---if they gave the go-ahead for an all out push this day, it is too late -- IT IS TOO LATE! YOU MUST HAVE HEROIC MEASURES AND YOU MUST HAVE THEM *NOW*!

For all of the reasons pointed out prior to this, your experimentation must go underground, underfunded, or out of the country entirely. How terribly unfortunate. Ones involved have already paid the ultimate price of being murdered and the remaining ones struggle on in full knowledge they are blatant targets. So be it--they will be given support.

I am going to interrupt this document at this point to give you information: GET THE STRECKER MEMORANDUM, ALL PROCEEDS ARE POURED BACK INTO THE RESEARCH--THE INFORMATION FOR OBTAINING THE MATERIAL WILL BE GIVEN IN THE BACK OF THIS DOCUMENT.

BLISS OR SUICIDE?

You all know it is easier for a king to have a lie believed than a beggar to spread the truth. WE are spreading the truth about AIDS for you are sitting helpless in your entangled web and you have prayed for help and this is your response.

Unfortunately, the truth is not pretty. The fact is you are not being told the truth by your government or the so-called AIDS experts who hold your very thread of life in their lies. Your media, for whatever reason, for they present all other heinous material--with advertising, will not present it to you. Of course they ridicule and poke fun at ones who commune and visualize our craft and we are all over out here in your spaces and many of our craft and murdered crew are in your prisons and military hangers. AH, TRUTH WILL ALWAYS OUT---SOONER OR LATER, IT WILL COME FORTH!

So you can choose to go right along with the official propaganda and play your fiddle while your "Rome" burns. These are the same ones who gave you brain cancer (SV-40 virus) as a result of contaminated polio vaccines in the early 1960s; a polio-like disease from their contaminated Swine Flue vaccine in the 1970s; and AIDS from their smallpox and hepatitis B vaccines; or, you can at least make yourself aware of the clear and present dangers that you all face----what is the price of ignorance? So be it.

Enough for today, Dharma. I am sorry to have to cause you to print such unpleasant information. Unfortunately, upon your blessed mother earth, there is little wondrous and pleasant information for it is the time of change.

I take my frequency to stand-by status that you might rest well and we shall proceed on the morrow. My colleagues await their opportunity to share.

SALU AND GOOD EVENING HATONN TO SIGN OUT

CHAPTER 8

REC. #1, HATONN

FRIDAY, OCTOBER 13, 1989 6:30 A.M. YEAR 3, DAY 058

Hatonn in the light of the Radiant One, Commander Immanuel Sananda. Are we ready to begin? Thank you.

It is fine, Dharma, Commander Ashtar is here and only wished to make a bit of a preface--we will leave it for tomorrow. What it concerns is technology as backup material for you ones that you might check out other things which are sidetracked and hidden from public view to secure jobs and status.

It deals with Constable's methods of environmental atmosphere control, specifically as utilized in Southern California to negate and drastically reduce pollution. Those studies were done a couple of years ago, a drastic reduction was documented, the results stolen and false reports were made public by the Air Control service itself.

Therefore, the group with the equipment re-ran the experiments this past year, ending in July. Again, drastic changes in smog warnings and pollution levels as reported---although pollution reports were continued on public media. This time, an independent, private screening service was employed for testing and the results were concluded and presented.

All available documents were again stolen, with harm to the bearer thereof. Ashtar will present those findings to you readers. The information is again being compiled at your physical level and when we know it is public "somewhere", we will give input. All ones must be constantly reminded--caution is uppermost for Dharma's security--we will not jeopardize her safety to give you ones a "scoop".

Pollution of the environment is a multibillion dollar business. A Mr. Merkel, of Texas, some fifteen years ago had a superb device already perfected and tested to remove the problem of acid rain. It was a relatively small device which would fit either into an automobile exhaust system or within the inside core of a smokestack which converted the polluting matter into battery acid for recovery and further use, and pure, distilled water. Do I need say more as to what happened to that wondrous plan? The device used polymers and silicon; was most simple in concept and very nearly "free" of expense. In fact, the byproduct of battery acid for electrical storage would have returned great profits in itself.

You ones had best stop arguing over whether or not the ones who control you would or would not do these things to you BECAUSE THEY DO--ALL DAY, EVERY DAY! Then they go change your constitution to disallow flag burning. What a gross distractor, it will only make it more meaningful to the flag burners to burn the symbol. You can regulate, by law, neither morality nor patriotism for that is individual and from within--you only place further

, on you the people. Your constitution was set up in perfection ı your forefathers and galactic ambassadors; you have torn it away ıce.

You are most fortunate for you remain a favored country wherefrom wondrous things are yet to come. So be it. Let us move back into our document subject for naught but downhill is your destiny if your people don't wake up and take notice of truth and climb beyond your imprisonment for you are losing of your freedoms hour by hour.

* * * * *

CAN AIDS TAKE A NATURAL COURSE AND DIE OUT?

NO! You ones are being told that heterosexuals need not worry at all, that the AIDS virus is a sexually transmitted disease, that it is not easily transmittable, and there is no evidence that it is spreading into the heterosexual population.

Dear ones, there are well over 75 million African heterosexuals infected according to your own World Health Organization. That is in all colors and creeds. The numbers are doubling every few months.

What are the acceptable scientific prerequisites for eradicability? Another quote here from one of your renowned virologists, Dr. Frank Fenner, Center for Resource in Environmental Studies in Australia. This is a medically accepted criteria:

Under prerequisites for eradicability, one can virtually rule out the possibility of worldwide eradication of an infectious disease if ANY ONE of the following criteria are obtained:

1. The agent grows in wild animals or birds." Therefore if you believe that it came from monkeys, which it did not; or, you believe it came via domesticated cattle and sheep, which it did, either would preclude eradicability.

2. "The infection persists in the affected human being for years in their recredences." These viruses exist for 14 years or longer, and, having a slow viral progression obviously makes the second factor for noneradicability.

3. "The disease has multiple serological types." There are thousands of variants to the AIDS virus; at least 9,000 to the fourth power, different AIDS viruses possible, which makes the third criteria voided.

4. "The necessary degree of social cooperation cannot be obtained, as with the human venereal diseases." In other words, if the disease is a sexually transmittable disease, or venereal disease, then you cannot eradicte it from humans once running, because you cannot obtain the degree of social cooperation necessary for eradication. And most certainly this category, true or false, is the mass perception and social cooperation is based on mass belief.

Therefore, not only does AIDS violate ONE of these criteria, as required above, it violates ALL FOUR!. Once you have AIDS running helter skelter among you in humans, you are destined to have it for a very long time or until it eradicates your species. You have a horrendous problem facing from all the mutations of the virus, not just the AIDS virus alone.

TREATMENT?

At the present time there is a drug being widely utilized for those who have the abundance to afford it, I believe you call it AZT. The virus will preferentially use this in its self creation which leads to a defect in virus production and the virus begins to die out within the body. Of course, this drug also causes the body to die off so it is much less than perfection.

There are other things which lend strength to the immune system and give some stand-off resistance to the disease attack but do nothing for the killing of the virus, such as heavy intake of various vitamins and minerals. These do not solve the problem but do give some degree of life quality and prolong life function.

There is one treatment which has been most effective but again, is not utilized by your orthodox physicians. In cases of Kapose's sarcoma leisions which have been "cultured", there are present spirochetes--the attacker in syphilis. Dear friends, that can be treated with penicilin--but NOT as you are using it in the U.S. It must be a water based penicillin given in mega-dosage. The emulsion based penicillin as utilized today does not allow the penicillin to pass through the membranes and reach the affecting "critter". AIDS, surprisingly enough, if ones of you in the scientific profession would look closely, could be called a tertiary syphilis and many ones could be given a longer lifestream by such intervention.

There is now another substance coming onto your scene which has great promise of assisting in stalling off the ultimate death disease. The substance can cross the cell membrane and react with the virus itself. As it is validated, information on new substances will be provided through the Pubulisher.

THERE IS A WAY

There is a technique which is already in practice and available for the aforementioned select few. It is tinkered around about here and there in one or two of your universities, Baylor in Texas, being one. But it is basically forbidden investigation, and goes without any funding resources. (That is the one criteria which should cause you to know it is feasible!!!!)

Let me first use an example: If you bombard a crystal container with a specific sound wave (tone) it will shatter from the pulse vibration impact. Now, if you are holding that lovely wine goblet in your hand at the time it shatters, the glass may cut your fingers but the sound wave will do *nothing to your hand*.

VIRUSES ARE *CRYSTALLINE* STRUCTURES AND THEY WILL RESPOND TO SPECIFIC SOUND FREQUENCY EXACTLY AS THAT GOBLET. THEY WILL EXPLODE. NOW IS THAT NOT QUITE QUAINT? PERHAPS YOU CAN "SING THEM TO DEATH". THAT MAY BE BIT SIMPLISTIC BUT NOT BY VERY MUCH---YOU ARE NEVER GOING TO GET THEM ALL IN ANY OTHER MANNER!

ROYAL RIFE, GREATEST INVENTOR SINCE TESLA

In the years between your mid-twenties and say, 1945, R. Royal Rife had developed a method whereby he could irradiate the little crystalline viruses with the specificly proper radio sound wave, and disrupt them without disrupting human tissue.

Orthodox doctors promptly say that is, of course, hogwash (or worse). Well, the next question for the "nonsense" crowd is to inquire as to whether or not they think you can destroy viruses with light or shake them to death? Ah so--next ask them what method do they use in the laboratories when "critters" are blown out their hoods when they are experimenting. WHAT THEY USE IS ULTRA VIOLET LIGHT WHICH IS NOTHING MORE THAN ELECTROMAGNETIC RADIATION OF A PROPER WAVE LENGTH.

Even on dense Earth, it is proven beyond anyone's misrepresentation, that electromagnetic radiation of a proper form can and will kill viruses.

Right out of the aforementioned Baylor University, came the public information that they had taken blood which was contaminated with herpes virus, with cytomegalovirus (which is a deadly thing in an organ transplant patient), and with AIDS virus. They irradiated the blood with laser light and showed that they could kill the virus without killing the cells. The cells were still viable but the viruses had been destroyed.

Now would that not somehow broach the very topic of *electromagnetic* cure of viral diseases? THIS, READERS, IS FROM WHENCE THE AIDS CURE WILL COME.

A simple machine, much more simple than your accepted x-ray equipment, can be utilized which will identify, based upon readings determining what kind of virus is present, and treat the human being with a frequency beam jolt which will destroy the virus contained within, not only his blood but throughout his entire body. It must be throughout the body to preclude reinvasion.

You can then eradicate, not only AIDS, but all other human retroviruses as well. They are nothing more than animal retroviruses running in humans. Persons can be cured individually and the diseases eradicated worldwide. You sure could clean up your animal herds as well.

WELL, WHERE IS DR. RIFE?

The virus is a very, very minute little beastie that is very hard to see by a means whatsoever. Dr. Rife devised a method whereby he could visualize the viruses. Rife was a most gifted machinist and invented a microscope with which he could actually view viruses in the living state. The microscope had a magnification of 70 to 100,000 times in living tissue. These machines existed in fact, and two or three are still around today just awaiting eager minds and hands to bring back into perfection. It requires a whole concept change of thought acceptance, however, from your scientific community---you see, things have not politically nor egotistically changed in mankind in those ensuing years.

Rife actually invented this machine and could view viruses in living tissue and also was able to determine the mortal ocillatory rate, which is the frequency with which he would irradiate the viruses in order to kill them. Just as I utilize a frequency to communicate with Dharma here, I could also tune it up and explode her head, body or the most minute foreign particulate from any cell. I, nor do my collegues, even toy with such things for we are not allowed, by cosmic law nor without full permission of participants, to intervene in any manner. This is why you don't have body snatchers from outer space. To break the cosmic laws brings a very bad penalty indeed.

To intervene in planetary human activities is very, very severe lawbreaking. We must await full invitation for intercedence or the situation would include severe impact on the outer space beyond your atmosphere. We can observe, visit, communicate, send ones and all sorts of things but we do not snatch you nor harm you in any way. If ones cause humans to do heinous crimes or commit crimes, it is through agreement of that human and through his own willing actions. It is as with the misunderstanding of hypnosis; one will never do, in a state of hypnosis, that which he would not be most capable of doing wide alert with a little hit or two of alcohol or drugs. Forget your old wives' tales---we of the cosmic realms are not a threat to you--*YOU ARE A THREAT TO YOU!*

Dr. Rife called the mortal ocillatory rate the MOR. He found that he could bombard the cell, devisualize all atoms save the virus and irradicate it with basically monochromatic light, which today you would refer to as laser light, the virus would "illumine", would absorb energy and emit energy allowing visualization, and then by increasing the amplitude of the energy input into the virus he could cause the virus to disrupt.

This is not only feasible, it is absolutely credible and workable.

It works on the same basis as visualization of our space craft--given the proper frequency adjusted to the margin of human visualization we can be seen---that is a severe slowing of our ocillatory rate---or, the raising of the human individual frequency rate to match ours. A little of both has to occur to get anyone levitated through light beams--our mode of transportation, other than mental frequency utilized for teleportation in great perceived travel distances. We move in a time warp which recognizes no time nor space. Therefore, we mfortable time in your density which, over a period of time s us to acquire confusion, memory loss, et cetera.

must, however, be elevated beyond the base human spector thought patterns before we can move this orb through r higher frequency--that means a lot will refuse to change e the "physical" transmutation as the Earth does her own cleansing and topography changing. You are most unbalanced on your axis and when natural phenomena begin, it will be incredible and not one thing will be left without change.

IT IS MOST SURELY PAST TIME THAT YOU ONES RECOGNIZE US AND SHARE WITH US FOR WE HAVE GREAT GIFTS TO BRING UNTO YOU AND THERE IS MUCH PREPARATION TO BE FULFILLED ON THIS PLANET. I DID NOT MAKE THE COSMIC, UNIVERSAL LAWS OF THE CREATION--I SIMPLY FULLY ABIDE WITHIN THOSE LAWS AND YOU ONES WILL LIKEWISE LEARN TO SO DO OR YOU WILL ANNIHILATE YOURSELVES. THE PROPHECIES OF ENDING CYCLES ARE NOT MYSTICAL, IT HAS SIMPLY COME FULL CIRCLE AND YOU ARE WITHIN THOSE CHANGING TIMES WHEREIN THE EARTH WILL CLEANSE HER-SELF AND THOSE OF YOU WHO WISH TO STAY AROUND AND PARTICIPATE WILL CLEAN UP YOUR INTENT AND ACTIONS---IT REMAINS YOUR FREE-WILL CHOICE WHICH IT WILL BE.

YOU WILL NOT BE ALLOWED TO BRING YOUR TOYS OF DESTRUCTION AND BEASTIALITY INTO OUR UNIVERSES TO UPSET THE ORDER OF THE SYSTEMS. SO BE IT FOR THIS IS THE LAW OF THE COSMOS AND YOU OF THE PRISON PLANETS WILL REHABILITATE YOURSELVES OR YOU WILL NOT BE ALLOWED TO PLAY WITH US.

Dharma, let us leave this please. Commander will discuss your hidden weapon systems of time reverse waves, what you call "scalar" waves, Tesla beams, etc. I remind you, chela, that it is not for your understanding, except in a most general way, that this information is being selected. There will be great meaning to ones who will receive of it in proper intent. Mr. Russell and Mr. Tesla remain in stand-by. As a Co-Commander and your cohan, I salute you for your service.

SALU, SALU, SALU---IN THE TRIUNE OF POWER I SERVE.

I AM COMMANDER GYEORGOS CERES HATONN

FREQUENCY CLEARED, HATONN TO SIGN-OFF

CHAPTER 9

REC. #1, HATONN

SATURDAY, OCTOBER 14, 1989 8:30 A.M. YEAR 3, DAY 059

Hatonn present to discuss current news before we move back into the subject of retroviruses.

I am going to "tell you so", little chela, then I am going to urge you to get SPIRAL TO ECONOMIC DISASTER into the public *last* month. While men fiddle the house of cards falls down.

To refresh your memories back over a year ago---we told you exactly how it would come to be, six months ago I told you to get out of the market and convert to all the cash in small bills which you can and bury if necessary. It told you the major signs, at least, and probably the market crash would come this fall of '89 and further, get this all finished before November----now what is it you don't understand, Dharma? I told you when we penned the document that it would be doubtful if we could print it in time---but, you see that was weeks and weeks ago. THE BIG BROTHERS DON'T WANT THE INFORMATION OUT THERE, CHELAS.

We could do a two thousand page document on every various circumstance in your country alone, much less the entire world and only boggle you. We effort at getting you information to make this transition in some form of physical "aliveness" so these dastardly things must be brought forth first, without much input of spiritual nature. As things prove to be correct so that man can "trust" our input, they will immediately recognize the Captain of the ship.

You ones are being eaten alive and have sold yourselves on the lie that it is for your own good and demand more and more and more control from your government; demand that your government take more and more money from you to foot the bill for those things you insist upon and just where do you "think" you will be when the chaff blows away? The ones who, let us say, burn your flag in protest are not your traitors--it is the ones who write and enforce new and heavier enslavement that are the traitors and you recognize them not.

WE RECOMMEND NAUGHT OTHER THAN INTELLIGENT OPEN MINDS TO ACCEPT TRUTH AND KNOWLEDGE. YOU MUST REALIZE THAT CIVIL CHAOS WOULD DESTROY YOU; SUBVERSIVE OVERTHROWMENT OF THE GOVERNMENT WOULD DEVASTATE YOUR CITIZENS. YOU SIMPLY NEED AN INFORMED PUBLIC WHO CAN SEE WHAT IS GOING ON UNDER THEIR NOSES AND BUILD A BETTER WAY TO GO RIGHT UP THROUGH IT--NOT BY VIOLENCE; SHOW A BETTER WAY! THE SERPENTS WILL DEVOUR THEMSELVES; EVIL WILL DEVASTATE ITSELF--RE-READ YOUR PROPHECIES; YOU HAVE COME THE

TWO THOUSAND YEARS! IT IS IN THE FINISHMENT! *YOU ARE IN THE BEGINNING!*

Yes it is going to be worse and Germain walks every step of the way with the business proposals and yet the force is not being focused in full intent for this transition and greed is being poked into each transaction---perhaps your team will better understand this day-----what do YOU think will have happened by Monday eve? WE HAVE THOUSANDS OF HOURS OF TAPES DEALING WITH THESE SUBJECTS AND THOUSANDS OF PAGES OF WRITING DEALING WITH THESE MATTERS----WHY DOES SOMEONE NOT PULL THEM FORTH? WHY DO YOU CONTINUE TO ASK AND ASK THE SAME QUESTIONS ANSWERED IN DETAIL MONTHS AGO? WILL YOU NEVER COME INTO BELIEVING OF US? SOMETIMES, I TOO, DO NOT KNOW WHY WE COME OR WHY WE EFFORT FOR IT WOULD APPEAR SO HOPELESS. THE TRUTH ALWAYS COMES FORTH BURIED BY THE FOOLISH DESCRIPTIONS AND LIES WHICH ARE PERPETRATED TO DISCOUNT OF IT AND YOU ONES CHOOSE TO BELIEVE THE *LIE.* SO BE IT, HOW HARD DO YOU HAVE TO BE HIT TO UNDERSTAND? I HAVE DONE HOURS AND HOURS ON THE MARKET ALONE AND MORE HOURS ON THE ECONOMY AS A WHOLE AND THE COLLAPSE WHICH MUST HAPPEN. NO, I SHALL NOT GIVE IT AGAIN---*YOU ONES GET BUSY AND PULL THAT INFORMATION FORTH AND DO NOT JUST UTILIZE THE NEW BOOK FOR IT IS NOT ALL WITHIN THOSE PAGES. IF YOU LOOK WITH UNDERSTANDING YOU CAN DISCERN ALMOST TO THE MINUTE THINGS WILL PRESENT THEMSELVES. YOU ONES PERUSE THE LESSONS AND PUT THEM ASIDE AS TOO MUCH--THEN AWAIT AND MOVE ON TO THE NEXT DAY'S INPUT---NO, NO, NO--THAT IS LIKE SCANNING A NEWSPAPER; I SPEAK OF KNOWLEDGE AND UNDERSTANDING THAT WHICH GOES ON ABOUT YOU--YOU DO NOT EVEN HEAR THE ANSWERS TO YOUR OWN PERSONAL QUESTIONS. SO BE IT FOR YOU ARE IN IT, BROTHERS, AND IT WILL BE AS IT WILL BE AND YOU WHO HAVE NOT LISTENED SHALL SUFFER JUST AS DOES EVERYONE WHO DENIES.*

Why is man not prepared? You have been given thousands and thousands of years to prepare---long further back than the Man from Galilee a short two thousand years ago. If you but had a good shelter system your brotherhood of citizens could endure all those elemental storms about your coasts and that which will tumble on you from the sky. Dear me, how much *WARNING* do you require?

HATONN IS NASTY THIS MORNING? NO, HATONN AND COMPATRIOTS ARE SIMPLY IRRITATED AND AGGRAVATED. SO BE IT.

Let us return to the subject of AIDS retrovirus plague. If you do not do something quickly, about this issue, you need not even concern about anything else.

REMEMBER SOMETHING MOST IMPORTANT, YOU ONES WHO *PRESUME* YOU ARE THE CHOSEN ONES OF GOD FOR THIS TRANSITION---THERE ARE BILLIONS OF PEOPLE ON YOUR PLANET AND HERE IS WHERE *FREE-WILL* CHOICES COME INTO PLAY. THE ONES WHO TRAVEL THROUGH THIS TRANSITION WITH THE MASTER AND THIS BLESSED CREATION OF EARTH--NEED NOT BE ANY OF YOU. *FAITH WITHOUT WORKS WILL NOT GET YOU THROUGH AND WORKS WITHOUT GOD'S GRACE WILL NOT DO IT.* EYES AND EARS BETTER BE COMING TO ATTENTION!

Now, a word of caution to you ones who would rush into this area to work with Dharma and Oberli---don't do it, or be very cautious if you even visit in their location. What you ones may feel is good intent to "help" and "serve" the Masters is very likely to cost one or the other of them, their very lives. They are under constant and continuing surveillance. Do not even remotely "think" of coming into their proximity for dwelling with them or plan on grand or great "psychic" readings or seminars, etc. If you must participate in group hoopla, go to those of our brothers who are in that business, please---PLEASE.

OURS IS TO PRESENT THE WORD UNTO THE PEOPLES IN ALL FORMATS. YES THERE WILL BE MAGNIFICENT JOBS AND PARTICIPATION IN THIS AREA BUT PRESENTLY WE EFFORT AT *NO PERSONAL EXPOSURE WHAT-SO-EVER*. BUSINESS MEETINGS AND PLANNING SESSIONS OF BASIC FORMAT MUST BE HANDLED OUTSIDE THIS LOCATION OR WITH AT LEAST ENOUGH FOREWARNING THAT WE CAN CONVENIENTLY DISRUPT SURVEILLANCE ELECTRONICS AND SCATTER ELECTROMAGNETIC SPY FREQUENCIES. YOU THINK I JEST? TRY ME! YOU WHO THINK YOU WILL JUST OVERRIDE HATONN'S REQUEST--BETTER LOOK FOR THOSE LITTLE GREMLINS WHO CONTROL YOUR LIFE WHILE YOU ARE MAKING OTHER PLANS! OUR INTENT IS TO KEEP THIS GROUP PHYSICALLY SAFE AND THE INFORMATION IN TRUTH, FLOWING. OUR DARK BROTHERS AND THEIR HANDY-MEN ARE FULLY AWARE, AND FRANKLY, I DESIRE THE ALREADY FAMILIAR ENEMY THAN THE NEW TROOPS WITH WHICH WE HAVE TO TAG AND MONITOR. IF YOU DO NOT UNDERSTAND THAT WHICH I SAY THEN YOU ARE AMONG THOSE STILL "SEARCHING" AND LOOKING FOR PROOF FOR YOUR BELIEF SYSTEM--*RETURN WHEN YOU HAVE FOUND YOUR TRUTH--DO NOT JEOPARDIZE OUR EARTH PLACEMENTS FOR THEY ARE ALREADY FINDING IT MOST DIFFICULT TO FUNCTION AMONG THE EARTH HUMANS. THEY ARE CUT OFF FROM THEIR HIGHER ABILITIES AND INCREDIBLE LIMITS OF KNOWLEDGE AND WHAT YOU ONES WOULD CALL "MAGIC" ABILITIES ARE FORBIDDEN THEM TO UTILIZE. THEY MUST FUNCTION ACCORDING TO INFORMATION THAT WE PRESENT THAT WE CAN MONITOR THAT WHICH YOU ONES OF THE POPULACE ARE ACCEPTING AND UTILIZING. PLEASE EFFORT AT UNDERSTANDING THE CIRCUMSTANCES OF NEED FOR CAUTION. THE MOST VALUABLE CONTRIBUTION ALL*

ONES CAN MAKE IS TO UTILIZE EVERY METHOD AVAILABLE TO GET THESE DOCUMENTS PUBLIC AND TO THE "BEST SELLER" LISTINGS---MAN MUST SEE THAT WHICH IS GOING ON ABOUT HIM---THE TIME TO "WAKE-UP" IS AT HAND!

Dharma, before Commander Ashtar moves on into an in-depth discussion of Prana (solar-cosmic; scalar--you ones have dubbed it) electromagnetics in generalized presentation, you will please spend the next few hours translating and transcribing "Paul Andrew's" last recordment. Thank you, chela. As a mother who lost the young man prematurely, it is a difficult task but it must be done for Paul carried many portions of great significance. We honor him for a job well done in the black density of your environment.

Yes, chela, I do want this portion placed within the AIDS document and made available to any who receive the portions as they are presented, for security.

Please call when you are ready to continue.

HATONN TO STAND-BY

CHAPTER 10

REC. #1, ASHTAR

SUNDAY, OCTOBER 15, 1989 8:00 A.M. YEAR 3, DAY 060

Good day. Ashtar to begin, please.

Most of the ones on your placement who are delving into the proper approach to retrovirus cures on your place, continue to relate it to war "beams", frequencies and thus and so. Yes, these things exist and should be spoken of, however, I do not wish to get into lengthy discussions of war machines except as relates to AIDS.

Suffice it to say, you keep trying to get massive receiving systems into space to receive and further disperse these weapons. You have mammoth problems for you cannot handle the accidents which occur. For instance, at Chernoble and the laboratories in Livermore, California.

These beam systems require mammoth amounts of power to make the projects feasible and, therefore, facilities are usually built very close to atomic plants or major electrical installations, i.e., your San Clemente system. This is your most deadly toy and, out of control, causes chain reactions which can pulverize your planet in a matter of seconds. You have no known method of controlling such a chain reaction. I will point out a few interventions, at Earth request, with which you can recall and relate and then we will move on with the subject.

The worst hazard is that the beam, itself, feeds upon itself and backfeeds along its own path right back into its source. At Chernoble this is exactly that which occurred. This also will give credence to the information Commander Hatonn has already given many times to you ones---we of the space command were asked to stop the reaction--we did so, but not until far too much damage had been done to quietly shut down the system without great penalty to both you and to the fleet craft.

You see, for one of our craft to get close enough to the source of the beam thrust, we must move into the electronic field which disables our stabilization controls. Once manifested into visible form we are a "mass" vulnerable as are you in human form. In December of 1988, space command was again summoned by the Soviets, and at this intervention we lost a Pleiadean craft with crew. Nine of the dozen or so crew members were killed outright and the remaining ones were severely burned and injured. The Soviets, however, treated our men with great respect, care and brotherhood. We sent in our own physicians and treated these crew members until they could be safely transported home. A second ship was sent to retrieve our people and it was a most appreciated action.

Again, just prior to your major summit meeting, there was to be just another little show of force to you ones and again they had a backfeed problem. We were again summoned for intervention, we responded and again we were disabled and our craft was brought down. This time, however, there was relatively minor damage and repairs were undertaken and we were able to salvage the craft.

Then at your own research lab, as mentioned above, you got a test completely out of control which blew your capacitors and transformers and headed for annihilation. We were called in by your government on this occasion and were, in fact, able to stop the reaction without loss of craft or crew. This was also in 1988 and was announced in your media as an electrical problem.

Oh yes, your leaders know us well, friends, very, very well. We have representatives, usually myself and Commander Hatonn, to all high level meetings--albeit in holographic format any more for you made a bad blunder of "capturing" us at one such meeting----we are higher forms of vibration and you cannot hold us---you <u>can</u> hold our manifested representatives of a bit lower dimensional format.

Why would we respond? Because these are the beams which will blast you into oblivion. You would become a mass of problem to the corners of the universe. We would at that point of explosion have massive atmospheric reaction about your planet that we could not stop. We would encapsulate your sphere within a plasmic shield and hope we could contain you enough to continue your orbit and lessen impact to your solar system. You, as man and civilization, would be vaporized.

We are not allowed to stop your little atomic-seek, find and destroy, war games; we are ordered to intervene in planetary annihilation situations.

All of this information has been abundantly given unto you ones in the hours of instructions and communications with ones on your placement. Dharma and group have thousands of hours of such, recorded in time segments of action at the time of the occurrence of the event--in minute detail. Someone must organize and pull forth in proper cataloging of information that we do not need repeat and restructure for you for we have no time for repetition. It does, however, require ones who are self-sufficient for there is not yet industry to support individuals.

This is the problem of you ones who go from place to place with lots of good intent and no means of support. The work and actions are backward. At the time of the Master in Galilee there were no facilities and therefore, the speakers went from place to place abiding and surviving from another's labors in exchange for the receiving of the word. Now ones appoint themselves to hop, skip and jump about at random bearing their perceived calling. You cannot reach the masses in that manner and it is all but useless, worse, it causes your brothers to ridicule and place you in a grouping perceived as drop-outs, hippies, leeches and worse. Just as Immanuel Jesus Sananda will appear in a uniform of space command instead of flowing robes of sack cloth, you ones must stop your foolish hogwash.

Ah yes, Commander Ashtar is severe and blunt----we of these realms KNOW how it is, you paint the pictures as you HOPE it might somehow be---and you dear ones, are on the very brink of total devastating, agonizing annihilation. Further, millions of your so-called "Christian" brothers will be waiting for some big "lift-off, up and away" into some glorious cloudbank and what will really happen is that they will turn us (the real thing) away and choose to go into the void with the dark brotherhood in their ignorance. GOD DOES NOT MAKE SLOPPY, DRIFT AROUND ON CLOUDS, PLANS. A PLACE IS PREPARED FOR EVERY ONE OF YOU AND YOU PLAY AT LET'S PRETEND GAMES. "LET US JUST PRETEND, CHANT, PRAY, HOLD HANDS, SING SONGS, WEAR WHITE, BLUE OR PURPLE AND MAYBE IT WILL ALL JUST GO AWAY!" IT WILL NOT GO AWAY. IT IS ALL COMING DOWN THE PIKE JUST AS EXPECTED AND WORSE THAN YOUR WILDEST IMAGINATION COULD CONJURE. OH, THERE WILL BE GLORY AND WONDROUS EXPERIENCE FOR THOSE WHO UNDERSTAND THE TRUTH OF IT BUT THOSE WHO BLIND THEIR EYES, PLUG THEIR EARS AND TURN GOD'S EMISSARIES AWAY WILL FIND THAT ANGEL LUCIFER HIMSELF, HAS BEEN PLOTTING THEIR PATH FOR THEM WHILE CONSTANTLY URGING ONES TO BELIEVE "WE" COME IN EVILNESS--NAY, BROTHER, WE ARE YOUR WAY OUT AND THAT IS THE TRUTH OF IT. IT TRULY IS NOT EXPECTED THAT VERY MANY, RELATIVELY, WILL RECOGNIZE THE TRUTH BEFORE IT IS TOO LATE.

Back to our subject with only one comment regarding your current "market" problem. Watch what happens now; the effort will be made to shore up the problem with a bit of plastic tape. Paper money will pour into mutual funds, etc. to effort at holding the line on withdrawals and cashouts. This will, if it works, place the funds in worse jeopardy. You are in a most precarious monetary mess. Pray, however, that it works for we need a bit more time prior to the overall collapse. We need major funding for our projects and we need a few more weeks to get that in order. Dear ones, please understand that YOU ARE IN IT! IT IS ALL ABOUT YOU NOW---YOU EITHER ACT ON THE INFORMATION WE BRING OR BE PREPARED TO PAY GREAT PENALTIES---GET OUR INFORMATION OUT THERE. GET THESE DOCUMENTS READ AND OUT TO THE MULTITUDES. DON'T TRY TO COPY THEM INDIVIDUALLY; GET A RESOURCE OR SEVERAL AND TELL PEOPLE WHERE TO OBTAIN THEM---WE ARE GIVING YOUR INSTRUCTIONS TO WALK OUR ONES THROUGH, AS MANY AS WILL HEAR AND WALK WITH US, THESE ENDING CYCLE CHANGES AND INTO, THROUGH AND BEYOND THE TRANSITION. SO BE IT, SO BE IT.

WHAT ABOUT AIDS?

You ones are facing a magnificent problem of mammoth proportion. It requires instant action and funding in large amounts, but because the workers are life motivated instead of greed motivated, surprisingly less than you might anticipate. We are prepared to divert any profits from these documents right back into the programs involved--therefore it would be good if ones would purchase the books or contribute directly to the research teams. This will never be supported by your government funds, whereas a shelter system might be, therefore, plan your input well and place assets in the most priority manner.

Only a handful of researchers are available who can do the work. You will be prevented from having the already developed hardware so prepare yourself for that aspect; don't expect it and you won't be left twiddling your fingers. When you have about perfected your machinery, the big boys will probably come forth so that they can again, "*save the day*". You have to keep in mind that the controlling few are very selected and most of your congressmen, et cetera, are as misled as are you. But to do anything in time to save the masses is out of the question, as your governments now function. Even working around the clock, you will still lose great numbers of lives to this plague and that is inevitable.

Proper electromagnetics is your only solution and it must be set up most quickly. You have had ones pass before this time and some within your format now, who have done the work. Drs. Tesla, Russell, Rife and Priore have done it, if only you will assess it carefully. You do, however, have to bring your current workers into a unit--Strecker, Cathie and others who are too much in danger to name in this document. I name these ones for they are already most public and already understand their jeopardized situation. Earth-man, you have many gallant and daringly brave ones who continue to work in your behalf in spite of the constant impending danger to their lives and those within their family units.

These documents would already be before you but ones continually fell away in fear and terror. TO LIVE AND WORK FOR A CAUSE, DEAR BROTHERS, IS FAR MORE PAINFUL AND DIFFICULT THAN TO DIE FOR A CAUSE. DEATH IS NAUGHT BUT CHANGE. PONDER IT, PLEASE.

Expanded prana electromagnetics can solve the problem if you dare get on with it. If you can pull your nucleus of knowledgeable researchers together, you can find thousands who can do all of the other support tasks, such as testing, control studies---all sorts of backup tasks.

MASTER CELLULAR COMMUNICATION SYSTEM

The intrinsic virtual state of cellular control has already been discovered and pointed out. This massive communication system controls all cells in a body and all the functions thereof. This is a "life electromagnetic" system. Your new researchers wish to call this system "Scalar", we have no objections, therefore, I will refer to this as SEM since you ones do enjoy your alphabet.

The SEM conductivity pattern is not through the electron shells of the atoms but is directly through the nuclei SEM pathways. The SEM pattern's organized signals, non-specific vector electromagnetic (EM) waves, which externally sum the zero vector on already existing waves, can be constructed for virtually any specific purpose. This includes the ability to destroy a particle such as a virus, cancer cell, leukemia, bacteria--anything within or without individual cells--these frequencies can be created which will actually alter the very DNA/RNA. Through this approach the immune system and repair system of the body or cell, itself, can be reached and manipulated selectively. Thus, the entire biochemistry and functioning of a cell, including its genetics, is totally engineerable.

Further, a specific "charge pattern" can be designed and utilized to charge up the nuclei of the biosystem to fabricate specific immunity response. This charge, once established, is then maintained by the "master" system to allow for permanent immunity--in other words, you change the master computer to include the new and reject the old data.

To understand this just stated concept, you need to know something about brain, mind and thought basic functioning. It has been isolated and described on your place sufficiently to scientifically organize it. It, of course, is crude in isolation for it is the etheric aspect of life itself and you ones are not given to understand it in actuality. The concept is sufficient for this discourse.

MIND AND THOUGHT DESCRIBED

You ones continue to search in difficult helter-skelter fashion to isolate something which is so simple you cannot find it. You look where it cannot be found. Search within the limits of where a thing can be found and since all life is electrical energy in one format or another, look there first. Look within the electrical system. Consider the ionic discharges in and across the tremendous numbers of synapses of the human nervous system--it is wondrously constructed by creator, and the slower discharge and migration of ions across cellular membranes. If you take it as a single biological ensemble, you will find these are much like a vast array of continual and ongoing spot discharge vectors, charged current vectors, et cetera. Overall, within the microscopic space occupied by the body, these electromagnetic vectors sum almost to entirely zero resultant. Now, don't let this throw you into confusion. This is a general explanation intended for ones who do understand it, to know they are on the correct path and give further insight while giving all of you an overall view of the whole. We, too, must unfortunately work in mysterious ways our wonders to perform---we are not allowed to "do it for you"!

Dharma, you will note that we speak here in terms of zero, non-zero, sub-zero and plus-zero. I would wish that you would relate this in concept to Paul's theories. And, yes, the tape you transcribed is not the final one as was given to you by him in March of '85. But it will suffice for the concept is correct and we shall ultimately give him credit for his contribution was of the ultimate physical separation. He shall be honored for that which he has given unto this mammoth cause for he was "out of his time" and for those blessed beings it is pure torment of inability to adjust or "fit-in". It requires those ones to stimulate actions of others into their accepted and intended tasks. I hope this helps you to understand, chela.

When I say that these electromagnetic vectors sum almost to entirely zero resultant, it is that only a tiny non-zero vector residue remains. However, this vector zero summation has incredibly rich enfolding signals and channels and dynamic relationships and structures within it.

This zero vector summation is the biopotential of the body whole. It is constantly and dynamically changing. For those of you who perceive in esoteric terms, this is the "auric" field---the aura. It has multiple virtual state levels, it is anchored in and resides within the atomic nuclei of the mass of the body. It is a virtual-state "engine" activating, structuring and dynamisizing the virtual particle flux of the charged particles of the body. Hence it is finely structured and controls the body's dynamic charges and charge distribution. This, then, is the fashion in which it controls and erects the body's biochemistry.

Dharma, I am being summoned and therefore request a break. Thank you.

Ashtar to stand-by status

CHAPTER 11

REC. #1, ASHTAR

TUESDAY, OCTOBER 17, 1989 7:00 A.M. YEAR 3, DAY 062

Ashtar present. I am requested to make comments regarding urgent matters.

Oberli, be aware that surveillance has been increased in your location. You will please ask "Victory" to relinquish direct contact with you to a minimum. Our wish is to exclude no-one from their contribution but he becomes a most watched and controversial person. Pre-information is now in the hands of top elite military personnel prematurely. It is through the slow production of the book that the plan is altered. It is what we wished to have happen but not until the SPACE-GATE was actually in public. We desire the government denial but not the slowing of distribution. These books must get into public hands; why is SPACE-GATE still not public? It has been in Sedona since August.

Worse still, in order to have a place of contact, the most damaging material of all time has ability to focus directly back to the scribe and all the precautions we have taken to keep her unknown are now instantly gone. Victory, in his exuberance, has drawn the enemy right into your very encampment. So be it, we will need increase protection and you must keep Dharma pretty close to home.

Ones are still at play; self oriented, drifting, experimenting and making themselves more publicly known--you ones must see and know, is why we have allowed it to happen, but there must come great self-discipline and control, with self-support to enter into this space for it is so very precarious for Dharma at this point. Love-ins and dream dancing are not the call of the day for you ones. Ones will NOT come into your space to dwell in tents and presumably "take care" of you. How foolish indeed. However, sometimes the foolish appearing jackal is more the wise master of the fox den---hold it in your heart. These ones in seemingly unwittedness mock the name of the Masters they claim to serve. We have great compassion and we have this incident under control---lessons are constant and unexpected. Do not badger yourselves over it for it has been guided. Ones who function without moderation are most dangerous to everyone. Each word spoken must be considered from the standpoint of its destination receiver. JUST A NOTE OF CAUTION, NOT A REPRIMAND, PLEASE. FOR WE NEED A COMPLETE SCATTER ON THIS INFORMATION AND I DO NOT WISH TO STALL YOU OUT--IT WAS GOING TO HAPPEN ANYWAY BUT THE FLOW BREAKDOWN CAME IN SEDONA. NEITHER IS THIS A REPRIMAND BUT ONLY ALLOWS YOU TO SEE WHAT A DIFFICULT THING IT IS TO WORK WITHIN THE BOUNDARIES OF FREE-WILL OF MAN. WE HAVE OUR PROBLEMS TOO!

DO NOT ALLOW IT TO BE GENERAL KNOWLEDGE AS TO WHERE ALL THIS PUBLISHING WILL BE COMING FROM. LET US

PROTECT THE RESOURCES. WE SHALL HAVE THEM OUT IN ABUNDANCE IN A MONTH SO LET US JUST MOVE RAPIDLY AND SILENTLY. DON'T BE OVERLY CONCERNED, JUST HEED UNDUE DANGERS. KEEP DHARMA OFF THE PHONE PLEASE, JUST ALLOW THE ANSWER MACHINE TO PICK UP MESSAGES IF ONES ARE NOT PRESENT FOR ANSWERING CALLS.

You will find that those vulnerable at top levels will do anything to cover bad leadership and management. Just as with the gun turret explosion on your U.S. ship (I name no names for I do not wish to further credit the lie), however, the elite have now dumped the blame of those deaths on a poor, blameless (and dead) sailor having now written the fiasco off to a suicide bomb placed by him, between ammunition storage. Evil knows no bounds, dear brothers, no bounds. It is just as with ones the enemy wishes to trap and get rid of, they will simply set-up a situation and place evidence or "whatever". You must leave them no opportunity to take note, and know that any radicals around you are the most closely watched. Dharma has no new information and the spies know it; add radicals running about and they will take her out one way or another. We monitor most exactingly what is given into these books that there is always backup known and available to those who do the surveillance. Just as with the shooting of President Kennedy by his bodyguard--the truth is in picture form all over your globe--you just did not happen to know it. We do not play with the lives of our scribes.

Enjoy the Nostradamus discourses. These are the way we are bringing forth updated material, through many ones at various levels of input. There will still be riddles which will only give information to a specific few but in general, all will have it along with final instructions. We will continually give you source information that is predominantly valid, that all ones can have access and give working funds and material to continue dispersement. Give information forth regarding the sources of our recommended reading, please.

Let us now return to our subject. Keep these communiques of daily matters within the chapters of the books for at this point it is the only way to get these messages to the many. As you move further, your publisher will be given information for continuing arrangements. You just go on about your business for as you are guided into the proper channels, you will be given relief from the massive burden. We see and understand the situation and remember, it takes time to lay groundwork for massive building, ones have to come into realization of their proper portions, etc., etc.

I believe we left off on the 15th in the middle of a dissertation on --

MIND AND THOUGHT FUNCTIONS

I was speaking of non-zero residue. Modern scientists consider this residue and try to ascertain where and how mind and thought are accomplished by the residue. No, that is the incorrect approach. The residue, the ENH field remainders, are simply garbage--waste. It is the engine operating inside the vector zero summation that must be considered. These exhaust by-products are not the functions of the mind/thought process itself but rather they are the spillage resulting from the function of the process itself.

If you put the mind into a state of rest and photograph the components of the zero vector summation, actually see the highly complex enfolded structure (pattern) of these components; then take a second "frozen" time photograph of the same components a very, very short time later, subtract the previous "frozen" pattern (the delta --"difference") between the two patterns represents the myriad of thoughts or specified forms in the virtual state. In a general sense, this represents the contents of the thinking mind. Each entity will have a varying thought pattern for each individual has relatively different thought impact from a given exact trigger thought point. But you will be able to understand better, the actual electrical circuitry of the function itself. Further, the speed from "normal" to "impaired"; "fully functional" to "retarded"; "normal" to "substance damaged" etc., can in fact, be ascertained and damaged circuit synapses isolated.

The mind is the overall functioning and changing of the entire pattern substructure and the ability of the organism to have such and do such. The ability of the organism to "do" such and such requires a couple more "nested" levels of virtual state, two or more higher dimensions which in essence has the same meaning. Basically all those electromagnetic component vectors are in, at least, the fifth dimension and therefore can be referred as higher dimensional or in some definitions, hyperdimensional. I personally do not like the term "hyper" for it denotes exaggeration or ballyhoo instead of "higher". But you will run into it often in Earth literature. "Supra" or even "super" would be a better designation.

HIGHER DIMENSIONAL

Every component driving the vectors themselves is higher dimensional. A thought is an "exact" change of a vocalized pattern. The thought must come prior to the vocalizing of the sounds which form the verbal thought. Except, in the case of direct "channeling" as with this scribe--the pre-thought is mine and she has no pre-thought about the contents. This is, however, a most significant proof of the status of "higher dimensional form at work", the "super/supra" consciousness. It goes beyond the subconscious level of function.

Most thoughts are totally without consciousness, multiple, simultaneous or parallel. A few could be considered serially ordered, singularly considered and processed--depending on the consciousness involved.

The subconscious mind is totally a parallel processor--bunches of thoughts at once. The conscious mind, on the other hand, is totally a serial processor; only one thought can be handled at a given instance. Most persons never reflect on this matter, that they can only perceive one single thought at a time in the conscious state.

In a healthy, alert state the conscious mind is so rapid that by habit, persons believe they perceive many things at once. However, what is occurring is that the conscious mind is perceiving only the ONE while the subconscious is intaking ALL data surrounding the thought, from the room, the clothes, the accent of the speaker, on and on ---, and running a continuous library.

Now, when the conscious mind regards the subconscious contents it sees something which has multiple meanings--at once. That is symbolism. The subconscious offers symbols which have many meanings in its effort to communicate an idea to the consciousness. Dreams are an excellent example---or even "daydreaming"---efforting to get an idea into the consciousness. Only the individual having the "dream" can actually analyze it for it is the most personal of personal. It may take the skilled "dream work" therapist to allow the consciousness to receive the projected thought, but beware of psychiatrists and psychologists who "INTERPRET" YOUR DREAMS FOR YOU---ONLY YOU ACTUALLY KNOW THE MEANING OF YOUR DREAMS AND THAT MEANING CAN BE BROUGHT FORTH, BUT ONLY BY YOURSELF.

Why do I go into this material? Because change and master function of the body, through the tiny-most cell, is controlled by the mind and thought. A confused mind will produce an infirm physical response; likewise, a clear mind can heal an infirm body by clearing any defects from the control system.

POTENTIAL IMPACT OF SEM WAVES

The potential lays at the SEM ability to penetrate the nuclei and actuate internal changes within the substructures (thoughts). The nuclei are in continual "charge up". The particles change their states; they charge up to their impressed potential, including the potential of each component of that impressed potential. Mind, thought and memory all reside in, and are recorded in, the atomic nuclei.

The biopotential of the dynamic mind uses "negative" energy and "negative" "time". SINCE THE NUCLEUS IS POSITIVELY CHARGED, POSITIVE ENERGY AND POSITIVE TIME ARE NEGATIVELY CHARGED CREATIONS. That is exactly what you get from photon interaction with the electron shells of the atom. Since it operates in negative time, the mind biopotential in negentrophy, it can restore order from disorder, or chaos.

In this manner, the life blueprint of the living organism can maintain order in the midst of the entropy (a measure of the unavailable energy in a closed thermodynamic system so related to the state of the system that a change in the measure varies with temperature in the ratio of the increment of heat taken in to the absolute temperature at which it is absorbed). This definition is given herein so that you can carefully consider temperature as an important component of "blasting" a specific particle, such as a virus. Further, keep in mind this additional definition of entropy: The measure of a disorder of a closed thermodynamic system in terms of a constant multiple of the natural logarithm of the probability of the occurrence of a particular molecular arrangement of the system that by suitable choice of a constant reduces to the measure of unavailable energy. The living organism must be able to maintain order in the normal physical components of the cells of the physical body. Since the "AIDS" virus and mutations thereof, alter the actual DNA in all cells of an infected body, the overall body must be cleared. I assume I make my point.

Thus, the functioning mind and biocontrol system--the master cellular communications system, the immune control system, the acquisition system and the repair control system, all reside in the nuclei in dynamically interacting pattern potentials, or pattern charges, complete with resonances and frequencies and et cetera.

ANTOINE PRIORE'S "MACHINE"

Priore constructed an electromagnetic treatment machine and demonstrated a close to 100 percent "kill" (cure) of all kinds of carcinomas, leukemias, etc., in thousands of laboratory tests utilizing animal forms. These tests were openly shared with American scientists as early as your 1960's. At the time of the research, the French government funded several millions of dollars for Dr. Priore's research.

Into a tube containing a plasma of mercury and neon gas (hold this combination in your hearts for Sir Russell will expand on this subject later), a pulsed 9.4 gigacycles wave modulated carrier frequency of 17 megacycles was introduced. These waves were produced by radio emitters and magnatrons in the presence of a 1,000 Gauss (the cgs `centimeter-gram-second' unit of magnetic induction equal to the magnetic flux density that will induce an electromotive force of one one-hundred millionth of a volt in each linear centimeter per second at right angles to a magnetic flux) magnetic field.

Dr. Priore exposed experimental animals to this magnetic field during irradiation and a mixture of waves, some seventeen or so, coming from the plasma tube and modulating and riding the magnetic field, passed through the animal's body. *Among other things, as plasma can convert a transverse wave to a longitudinal wave, also phase conjugate, time reversal waves can be produced.*

Phase conjugated electromagnetic waves carry negative energy and negative time. They exhibit negentropy and move from disorder back to order. The proof is already in the hundreds of technical papers in non-linear phase conjugate optics in the orthodox scientific literature but ones continue to misinterpret the true definitions of terminology. Dr. Priore's apparatus produced a SEM signal with deliberately constructed, unfolded components including phase and conjugated electromagnetic waves.

Further, keep in mind that just to send out waves is inconsequential unless you have a correctly tuned receiver crystal for exacting frequency. You must integrate the information into a single functioning apparatus.

Dharma, I request a break at this time as I have other pressing appointments. I would like to cover some discussion of Dr. Rife's material today, however. Thank you for your attention. I understand that this is a most difficult task for you in that you must work without any technical knowledge. Trust that this information is of great value to those working on this project. In your service, I move to stand-by.

Commander Ashtar clearing frequency.

CHAPTER 12

REC. #2, ASHTAR

TUESDAY, OCTOBER 17, 1989 5:15 P.M. YEAR 3, DAY 062

5:04 P.M.: EARTHQUAKE IN SAN FRANCISCO

Yes, Dharma, Ashtar present. Let us not comment too greatly on the earthquake; I do request you keep close watch for within the past week you have had heavy quakes off of Alaska and Japan--it means the earth is in increased pressure around the plates. We don't seem to be able to urge you severely enough to get your attention--when those plates really slip it is going to be something beyond your belief and very few take action or plan for survival modes. So be it. It is not evacuation time yet so if ones expect to be doodled up into dandy space ships--it is premature planning! This subject has been covered most carefully and explicitly by Commander Hatonn--some of you really like to live on the edge--well, along that coastline is going to be a very big, deep edge any day now. Rest well and pray a lot, you who dwell on the brink. Further, any slippage on any major intersecting faultline can tip it all.

ROYAL R. RIFE

Back to our subject of AIDS and other retroviruses.

Royal Rife's work clearly demonstrated specific frequencies associated with particular viruses and disease organisms. In addition, his universal microscope, using evanescent waves, or waves with only hyperdimensional components, had no wave length limitations on its resolution. Consequently, it could see directly into the virtuous state past the limit of the photon. Indeed, it could not only see the exceedingly small point cells that lie between ordinary cells and are just barely visible to the "best" orthodox light microscope, but it allowed visualization of some sixteen internested, deeper and smaller levels of structures within the point cell. Nothing before or since has achieved such a penetration. There are two or three of these scopes around that can be brought into repair.

Using this microscope he could see virtual state energy forces functioning and moving. The biology his microscope revealed was far beyond the state of biology today. It was unorthodox in conception and presented a great threat to your orthodox medical and scientific communities. If you are going to create and spread an incurable disease to fit your purposes you most certainly do not desire the cure to get there prior to the infection. Oh yes, that is exactly what occurred, little dreamers. With his scope, Rife could not only "see" the little varmints but he learned to manipulate and control the living internal structure of living electricity. Now please refer to the Nobel prize this

..st week for the ability to isolate a single unit of electricity and stabilize it. Honors be to that one. Learn what you can from that researcher---you are going to find that electricity units are living structures.

Since internested levels of virtual state are also "higher" spaces, or hyperdimensional, Rife's microscope was the first and only instrument to allow vision directly into higher dimensions and observe the higher dimensional living forms.

In Rife's time such a thing was unthinkable to medical science, yet today with substantial evanescent wave technology already utilized in wave guides and with a well developed body of evanescent wave theory, you could prove that Rife's microscope was capable of doing precisely what he and other scientists reported. But what happens? It is further hidden to cover the lack of interest and ridicule of the past actions. Perhaps nothing in history ever changes except the names and places.

It is important to note here for the less sophisticated reader: "evanescent" means to dissipate like vapor--tending to vanish like a vapor.

Before I go further I will return to the phase conjugate waves and phase conjugate replicas of ordinary waves and signals. I have a tendency to move too rapidly even for my secretary and I apologize, Dharma.

Included in those exceedingly complex modulations and spectrums, every cell has a complicated electromagnetic radiation spectrum. An abnormal cell has an abnormal change to that spectrum. If you subtract the normal cell spectrum from the abnormal cell spectrum you have a specific delta that then, introduced into a normal cell, will convert that kind of abnormal cell.

When you have such a single pattern for cancer conversion, for example, you can irradiate a normal cell with it and turn that cell into a cancer cell. However, suppose you phase conjugate that cancer conversion single pattern. The phase conjugate replica will be the pattern that precisely converts that sort of cancer cell back to a normal status. With phase conjugate replicas of cancer cells specific delta frequencies are fed into the cells of a body having that cancer, the cancer cell's master cellular control system will modulate with these time reverse specific signals. That will return the cancer cells within the body to the proper master cellular control system of the animal.

Thusly, the cancerous cells will be immediately destroyed or reverted back to a normal cell. A very similar process exists for just about every disease bacteria and infectious agent, including the viruses of AIDS. As a matter of fact, the viruses are more easily disrupted due to their crystalline formation.

In the Soviet Union it has been proven that any cellular death and disease pattern can be induced by a specific pattern carried on an electromagnetic signal. If the target cells are bombarded with the pattern carrying carrier signals for enough length of time.

In Australia these experiments have been fully replicated and extended. These documents should be easily obtained, say by Cathie of New Zealand,

and nab onto the researchers. In Australia they have induced cellular death and diseases between cell cultures at a distance of over a hundred feet--a most convenient distance indeed. Unfortunately, these experiments-thousands of them, were done in military institutes; but I see no particular problem in obtaining them.

Scientists in West Germany have also replicated these cellular experiments. However, the important missing link is that these experiments have some unpublished data to be gathered; that portion was the corresponding Soviet work showing electromagnetic REVERSAL of cellular death and diseases conditioned by irradiation by phase conjugate replicas of the pattern carrying induction signal. Briefly: If an action in forward time induces a condition then the time reversal of that action will reverse the condition. *(YOU SEE, YOU ARE DEALING IN HIGHER DIMENSIONS WHERE THERE IS NO SUCH THING AS TIME AND SPACE!)* The concept is so laughably simple that it eludes you ones. The time reversal of an electromagnetic disease process is a specific electromagnetic healing process for that particular disease.

This is exactly the technique under intense research by the group mentioned by Commander Hatonn in preceding discussion in this book. You can develop a cure for AIDS along with a cure for cancers, leukemias and just about every other disease known to man--you can even clear those blocked passages in the circulatory system.

A BIT ABOUT PRIORE'S EQUIPMENT

In his device, Priore internally structured the carrier photons themselves, making them vacuum engines. This structure contained the dynamic delta for the disease. By introducing these spectrum to a giant rotating plasma he then phase conjugated his vacuum engines and then passed these time reversed vacuum engines down and through a strong magnetic field which thoroughly penetrated all cells of the biological organism being treated. The scalar components that are the structured photons representing the time reversal of the disease were absorbed and re-radiated in all cells, charging up the nuclei of the atoms and organisms to some potential level of that exact healing and reversing pattern.

In that way he passed a specific cancer reversal phase conjugate replica into every cell of the body, charging the cellular biopotential and producing a permanent healing delta onto the body's cellular master control system. In the process that cancels that in leukemia pattern, charging the nuclei was cancelled and discharged. The new time reverse charge also destroyed the cancer cells or converted them back into normal cells. That, my friends, cured the disease even in terminal instances---all of them. Yes, I said ALL OF THEM!

Further, for the disbeliever; he could cure sleeping sickness and any viral disease, et cetera, et cetera. In other words, the process represented a severe stress against any cellular control system delta encountered. This caused a return to the normal cell's and master cell's cellular control system of the body.

BUT WHAT HAPPENS TO THE NORMAL CELL WHO HAPPENS TO BE THERE?

Encountering the normal control system in normal cells there was no delta--therefore there was zero stress. Encountering the abnormal control system in tumor cells it produced great and specific stress on it and reverted it to the normal control system of the body's normal cell. If the cancer cell could not withstand the stress it died promptly. Thus, to a normal cell the Priore signal pattern acted somewhat soothingly as a stroking to normal cell structures and no interference occurred with the normal cell---that is, one whose scalar control pattern is locked to the body's master cellular control system and in phase with it.

The Priore signal stimulated and stroked the normal cell but did not injure it in any manner. On the other hand, the scalar potential pattern in and of an abnormal, say cancerous cell, is out of phase with the body's master cellular control system and is not phase locked to it. Hence the Priore signal causes direct interference with the abnormal cell's independent scalar control system. The interference pattern constituted the reconstruction of normal energy directed to the cancer cell and also jammed its abnormal scalar life signals. This destroyed the cancerous cell by two mechanisms: 1. Physical energy was channeled directly into the abnormal cells causing direct mechanical damage, and, 2. The cancer cell, being an independent living "critter", had its scalar life-channel connected to his primitive mind which connected his primitive mind to his body, jammed and terminated.

ABNORMAL RETURNED TO NORMAL

If the cancer cell was reverted to a normal cell by the Priore stress before being destroyed, it became just a normal cell and the Priore stress had no further effect upon it. Any disease with cellular, biochemical or genetic basis can be cured in like manner. Priore's method, for example, was clearly shown to be able to completely reverse fatty deposit clogged arteries and further, lowered cholesterol levels to normal even in the occurrence of abnormally high cholesterol diets.

Every cell of the body, however, even the hair must be irradiated and treated, that is, charged up with the signal for the disease pattern is located in *every* body cell. The master cellular control system is holographic. The pattern that is substructured and potential with its dynamic and oscillating component is in each component, that is, in each atomic nucleus, hence is in each and every cell.

Every structural level of the body larger than a cell also has its own correlated pattern of modulation on the overall. The biological organism can regenerate lost limbs, for example, if it can utilize its natural recovery process in a Priore manner. Even though Priore's work was presented to the French Academy of Sciences, it was far beyond the group's ability to understand the device or its function.

Friends, I do not speak of ancient history--I speak of the 1970s. The academicians knew nothing of scalar electromagnetics and phase conjugation and that is exactly what the Priore device was. More the medical world saw a phasing out of their very expensive services--a dual motivation to squash this unsettling crazy man.

Sad for mankind, in 1974 the funding was withdrawn just as Priore was completing a device which could irradiate an entire human body. It would have been capable of curing almost all human diseases. Ah, but then, you might not have been able to enjoy this plague and tribulation and the cycle ending would undoubtedly have been postponed. Man, unfortunately, rarely changes the probabilities in a positive way--just runs headlong into disaster faster and faster.

In that particular machine Priore utilized a lamp, in which 17 specific frequencies were mixed and modulated upon a 9.4 gigacycles carrier. The machine was large enough to irradiate humans over their whole body. It should have been capable of curing cancer, leukemia and AIDS in two, five minute irradiations--a week apart.

While Priore was still in your dimension (physically alive), a major thrust was made to bring the device to market and into medical research and into utilization. The devices were to be assembled in France and then shipped to purchasers, who would be large research and development laboratories where they could be brought into local specifications. I think it is sufficient to note that "big brother" put a stop to the funding for the project and the work had to be shelved.

It is a fact that such signals can reverse nearly every cellular illness or condition of the body. The program to produce the cure for AIDS in this manner only requires the necessary funding and the assembling of the persons (left un-named for obvious reasons) to do the job.

WHAT ABOUT THOSE SOVIETS?

Well, the Soviets proved conclusively that any cellular disease or death pattern can be transmitted electromagnetically and induced in target cells absorbing the radiation. They also found they could do this from great distances of some several thousands of miles. Do your cells cringe every now and then?

The Soviets reported their effect using near ultra violet photons as carriers. The ultra violet photons were those emitted in death by a diseased or damaged cell as it dies. That is the bioluminescence which carry the property substructure. Photon bombardment of the target cell culture by the death pattern photons, and remember these conditioned photons are specific vacuum engines, induced the exact disease pattern in those shells after a charge-up of kindred period of time. During that charge-up time the atomic model in a target cell culture was charged-up with tailored photon vacuum engines which carried the exact cellular death pattern. As charge-up proceeded, the death pattern was gradually introduced onto the master cellular control system, at the cells in the target culture.

The West German scientists utilized infra red waves, that is, the infra red conditioning photon vacuum engine. Please, particularly note that it is already well known in quantum mechanics, better known as electrodynamics perhaps, that when a photon is emitted from the surface of dielectric body, the entire dielectric body participates in that emission. *Another definition please: "dielectric": A non-conductor of direct electric current. Also, "dielectric heating": The rapid and uniform heating throughout a non-conducting material by means of a high-frequency electromagnetic field. (He who has eyes, please let him see!)* If a photon is absorbed on the surface of the dielectric body the entire dielectric body participates in that absorption. Note also, that whether or not cellular disease conditions can be corrected by time reverse signals must certainly have occurred to your friendly Soviets, since this has already been widely utilized in the Soviet's giant Scalar Electromagnetic weapons---oh yes, the same ones that backfeed.

THE BEAUTY OF RIFE

Rife's microscope could easily allow visualization of viruses for it could easily defeat the wave length limitation of the light frequency utilized.

It has now been proven, in your own physics studies, that the wave length limit in optical instruments can be violated by utilizing evanescence complex waves. Rife's microscope utilized such waves and thusly, normal light wave length was not a limitation.

When an instrument is utilized to make complex waves, it can also be utilized to make phase conjugate waves. Rife's microscope could also be utilized to determine the exact color frequency pattern associated with specific disease organisms. There is great knowledge herein for it allows for the exact matching of frequency patterns.

Well, Rife got the usual warm treatment by his fellow man in payment for his services. He was bound over into prison and when he was later released he was a broken and discouraged man. He lived out his remaining life in retreat and his death was hardly noted.

You are fortunate if you can act quickly enough, for there are ones still living who have direct knowledge of the workings of the scopes. If you get busy you can recover and replicate the work. If you tarry your population will be devastated by the plague called AIDS and you will find no open space large enough to spread your memorial quilt.

Dharma, it is late and we are both weary. Please let us close this and we will make our enemies on the morrow. In loving care and appreciation, I move to stand-by.

Commander Antheose Xandeau Ashtar to clear frequency.

Good evening,

Ashtar to out

CHAPTER 13

REC. #1, HATONN

WEDNESDAY, OCTOBER 18, 1989 7:00 A.M. YEAR 3, DAY 063

7.0 EARTHQUAKE IN SAN FRANCISCO, 5:04 P.M. OCTOBER 17TH

EPICENTER: SANTA CRUZ, CALIF.

Hatonn present, Dharma. I will make a brief statement about your current affairs; however, the questions and petitions coming forth are a bit annoying, even if understandable. Further, I see we will not get on with our work if we do not comment.

We are always amused in the midst of disaster to see the mind and mouth of man at work. Not one public statement has gone forth to say how fortunate that God set it up to change the fewest possible physical life-streams in the Earthquake area.

I will point out several things and I desire you ponder them most carefully as to how "accidental" it could have been.

1. How often do you have a world series baseball game played at 5:00 p.m. in one area? My scanners show not one death in that stadium filled to overflowing with people who would have been at work or moving homeward. Further, great numbers in the ballpark would have been killed in their isolated dwelling places or business places.

2. Most businesses closed mid-afternoon so employees could make it to their homes to celebrate the opening of the game at 5:00 p.m. which lessened the traffic on the roadways at the time of the quake.

GOD AND THE CREATION ARE VERY MERCIFUL TO YOU CHILDREN WHO REFUSE TO LISTEN. AND NOW, YOU ONES ON THE OTHER END OF THE FAULT LINE PETITION TO SEE HOW MUCH MORE TIME YOU HAVE! WELL, YOU AREN'T GOING TO GET THE RESPONSE YOU WANT--IT IS NOT FOR US TO GIVE IN EXACTNESS. HOW MANY WILL CONSIDER THIS A WARNING? ALREADY ONES ARE SAYING, "WHEW, WELL I AM JUST GLAD TO HAVE IT OVER WITH SO WE DON'T HAVE TO WORRY ANY MORE!" YOU HAVE BEEN TOLD TO EXPECT A PLUS 10 QUAKE THE LENGTH OF THE FAULT LINE---THIS WAS *NOT* IT, BROTHERS.

Warning--warning-warning! How many listen to warnings? Further, how many are relishing this happening and expect the bus from up here--the cloudbank with the Master? Could the Revelations be true, they ask? Is it possible this is the time? Get out your little calculators and figure it out!

Oh no, it won't be as you petition it to be---"let us know ten minutes before a problem" so "then I can believe". You have been warned, warned and warned again. We have even pulled ones out of this very shock area only to have them change their minds about truth and move to even more dangerous ground in the very affected area. So be it, I remind you----: "I shall come unexpected as a thief in the night." and "These things will come without warning. . . .!" No, you who work with me have protection but not in the face of forewarning--that is called free-will choice to be where you choose to be.

Evacuation? You could not believe how many life forms we have aboard ship this day--most have changed dimensions and are in a state of shock but we are most busy at our task.

Now, let me tell you something to ponder. Probabilities and "signs" are confusing---getting prepared is quite simple. Your seers saw this coming on October 18th--that is pretty close--you were off only by one year! In a realm of no time or space, that is pretty accurate. Many of you also "feel" changes and "something big coming down" this October and have voiced it----YOU ARE <u>NOT</u> GIVEN TO KNOW FOR MAN WOULD NOT AVOID DISASTER; MAN WOULD MAKE SURE THE WORST COMES OFF IN TIMELY FASHION.

How many disasters can your government's pocket books carry? You may be in line to find out.

DOES ANYONE HAVE YOUR RADIO TUNED TO MY STATION? HEAR ME--THE COASTAL AREAS OF CALIFORNIA, U.S.A. WILL FALL INTO RUBBLE---SOON! GET YOUR LITTLE SELVES OUT OF THAT AREA--NOW, POST-HASTE, OR RUN YOUR CHANCES, WE ARE CAUSED MORE AND MORE TO RELEASE ANY SUPPORT SYSTEM TO THE EARTH ORB AND ALLOW NATURAL UPHEAVAL. YOU WHO BELIEVE WE COME IN HOSTILITY AND EVIL INTENT BETTER CHECK YOUR FINGERS AND TOES, HEARTS AND BRAINS FOR I FEAR MOST OF YOU IN THOSE AREAS OF LOCATION HAVE LOST PORTIONS OF YOUR BRAINS.

Yes, you in Tehachapi will be hit also--I have never told you otherwise; I have told you that you of ours, will be secure and the area protected in a lift off if necessary to preserve the crystal. A 1,200 to 12,000 foot raise-shift is not be sneezed at dear ones--Father has not promised you a rose garden--you have been told it will be beyond your ability to comprehend.

<u>*YOU ARE BEING WARNED AS GENTLY AS POSSIBLE AS TO THE SEVERITY OF WHAT IS COMING FORTH---WHO WILL HEAR THE CALL? THE FATHER WILL HOLD AND ALLOW ALL WHO WILL COME TO MAKE THE TRANSITION IN PHYSICAL FORMAT IN ORDER TO CONTINUE YOUR JOURNEYS--IT IS MAN WHO INSISTS ON SEPARATION, NOT THE FATHER.*</u>

Dharma, let it be known herein that all ones along the coastal area cities are in grave danger of loss of both life and resources. We do not wish the machinery and "inventions" to be brought forth in those dangerous areas. What have we accomplished if, let us say, we see to it that Dr. Strecker completes his task and the Priore/Rife/Tesla apparatus is all finished and it all collapses down around Dr. Strecker's head and kills all the researchers---how foolish indeed. We desire funding come forth and we desire it to be funneled into the area of Tehachapi where we can see to its development and tending.

The same with banking of incoming funds--get them tended into banks outside the major disaster projected areas. You ones must get funds in money format to work on these projects--the system cannot bear much more of a load, it teeters on collapse already. Ones involved in funding have a last window to reap grand rewards and if you do not handle it well you will promptly lose it all back into the fall of the system---DIVERT IT INTO PROJECTS WHICH WILL RENEW YOUR LANDS AND PEOPLES---THE DISASTERS OF MAN AND GOD SHALL INCREASE UNTIL YOU WILL PLEAD FOR THE MOUNTAINS TO FALL UPON YOU THAT YOU MIGHT ESCAPE-----THERE SHALL BE NO ESCAPING. HAVE I NOT JUST INFORMED YOU THAT OUR SHIPS ARE TENDING MANY DEPARTED AND SEPARATED SOULS? WELL, THEY WOULD NOT BE ABOARD CRAFT IF IT WERE INTENDED THEY "ESCAPE". *NO MAN SHALL ESCAPE THE CHANGING OF THE CYCLE! SO BE IT AND SELAH! NO MAN SHALL ESCAPE SO HE WHO IS PREPARED (READ YOUR BIBLES AND LOOK CLOSELY AT THE SMALL PRINT AND THAT PORTION WHICH YOUR LEARNED ONES HAVE REMOVED)---NO MAN SHALL ESCAPE!*

Further, you ones who have impact and was given responsibility to see to the instructions shall be in the remembering of your commitments or you shall be caught in the quicksand where you bury your heads. Mine ones shall be lifted unto the craft for their work is done, the word is being sent forth as requested and ones who are "listed" are receiving--what you do with it is your concern, not mine. It is upon your head if you fail to tend the Father's flocks and turn to unwise greed and delays.

I want all of you to purchase this week's Time issue. The temple of the Jews will be rebuilt and Austria will come into the coalition, while THREE countries shall be integrated into other whole or removed--that adds to TEN! The plagues, famines, pestilence, wars and earth upheavals shall increase and be compounded. What more do you ones need as warning?

Doom and gloom Hatonn. Do you think I enjoy doom and gloom? Do you perceive I enjoy seeing my brothers in pain, sorrow and mourning? We come to bring you home unto the place the Master has provided and prepared for you in the Father's realms--in safety, love and joy. The doom and gloom is for those of evil and those who will refuse to hear the clarion call to attention.

You are in the days of compounding chaos wherein man will find himself well beyond his level of incompetence. So be it; let him who has eyes to see--see, and ears to hear--hear, for the day of the Lord is at hand and man shall be given to recognize both his weakness and his strength.

Commander Ashtar gave you warning to be alert in these current days--pay attention to all natural actions along the regions of your "ring-of-fire" and connect them for therein lies your greatest signals. Listen to God speak, not your earth humans who give "expert" edicts---those experts have told you UFO's don't exist, AIDS is not a problem, you don't need a shelter or survival program---sure would be handy for a few people in California this morning to have some emergency rations, cooking facilities, flashlights and nice cozy well constructed shelters for if you can remain in good health, man can rebuild. You have a problem in the water supply for in some areas gasoline is flowing in your storm drains---prepare and you can sustain yourselves. Let this lecture suffice please.

Dharma, I am in your service, as petitions come forth I shall respond. It is, however, most urgent that you get on with the virus material---PAY ATTENTION TO YOUR OWN INNER INTUITION SYSTEM--THOUSANDS KNEW THIS QUAKE WAS COMING TO THE MINUTE AND THOUSANDS KNOW EXACTLY WHEN THE NEXT WILL COME---YOUR ATTUNEMENT IS BEING SHARPENED, LISTEN TO YOUR OWN KNOWING--HEAR YOUR GUIDES FOR THEY NEVER LEAVE OF YOU--NEVER!

The pressure is beginning to crumble the Russian empire--don't miss these things covered by the distractions. Honnacker's extraction in East Germany is a major note for this date. Major indeed.

The public, and more especially the "secret" meeting between hated enemies in the Middle East is of major importance in ways you do not even see for there is no comment regarding the real issues being bonded. When that temple starts going up and the sacrificial rituals are totally reinstated within the citadels; beware, for the moment will be upon you. Now, how much more do you desire to know?

Go, please, for a break that we might get on with the instructions from Ashtar and the beloved scientists, Dharma. Go in peace, child, and give no thought to the cares of the day for you are in the Father's wings and we have note of you and yours--our ones are blessed and should rejoice in the moment for this is your purpose and your fulfillment. It is so and let it be recognized for that truth which it is.

Continue to look unto the heavens from whence comes your proof and reassurance--watch for our spectrum strobes for those are your "visible" connection to your various mother crafts, set to your frequencies--pay attention to all "nudges" and respond after clearing of your areas. Do not sit around speculating which is which and what and who--at this point it matters not and is only distracting from that which must be done.

The time has arrived and passed, we have renamed our central command craft "PHOENIX" and appropriate ones are permanently locked on to our system. Welcome aboard!

HATONN TO STAND-BY

CHAPTER 14

REC. #2, ASHTAR

WEDNESDAY, OCTOBER 18, 1989 10:00 A.M. YEAR 3, DAY 063

Ashtar present and ready for AIDS, greetings and blessings on the truth as it flows and may it find its intended receivers. I dictate, you write and God willing, prepared ears and eyes will receive. You were told that you would not understand that which would be brought by the silver cloud cadets and our intent is that just one receive a portion of insight from each subject and then in working together you will find the whole. I do not like working in the form of riddles either, but there is no choice for your controlling elements will stop at nothing to stop your completion of this material.

Your researchers are so very close to the answers that the sum is lost in the simplicity. So be it that Dr. Russell is available now for a bit of basic discussion, would you please receive.

SIR WALTER RUSSELL

Ah but would old friends, such as we, recognize the modern labels they tag upon our beings. Good day in the light and radiance of the whole. I would tarry and share in comfortable visitation but we have a most urgent task at hand which needs attention. We travel back a very long ways, my friend, and I am pleased to again be in the ability to work with you. Thank you for attending for I do not utilize the gift of ethereal writing.

How little man actually knows and understands; those bits and pieces of a magnificent puzzle which teases the brains and remains ever elusive to the grasping mind. For instance, no one upon your planes recognized how it is that crystals, as a simple example, get their various shapes--they are all "cube" fragments you must realize. How are they determined? Well, they are determined in space by the shapes of the "wave" fields which bound the various elemental structures.

Nor, in the end of the lectures and speculations, do you actually have much conception of what constitutes the life principle, nor the principle of growth and to cause disruption by "ungrowth" or disintegration? You must have a concept of the life principle spiral and ever cycling movement on frequency paths. You must know that there is a simultaneous unfoldment-refoldment principle which repeats all patterns in Nature sequentially and records and voids them as they are repeated. This is a most basic point of truth in that which you set out to do in the interruption of the life-streams of retroviruses---the case currently in point.

You must be aware of that recording principle by means of which the Creator carries forth the sum totals of ever sequential cycle in His unfolding and refolding universe unto the very end of its manifestations upon one planet and its beginning on a new one. Dear ones, this is far more important than casual "maybe so" and "maybe not". Again, everything--EVERYTHING--is a cycle of unfolding and refolding and I shall enlarge upon that concept more relatively a bit farther on in this documentation.

Within the secret which is "light" is the answer to *ALL* of these heretofore unanswered questions, and many more that you shall rejoice in the discovery thereof as you move along your path; those which the ages have not yet allowed to be in the solving. This revelation of the nature of light will be the inheritance of man in this coming age of greater comprehension. Its unfoldment will prove the existence of God as well, those acceptable even to the sciences and religions alike. That alone would be well worth this effort; would it not?

There is no department of life which will not be vitally affected by this new knowledge of the nature of Light, from the university to the laboratory, from government to industry, and from nation to nation. I simply find it difficult to present it all here in a hodge podge format of deletions to fit the urgent need. Therefore I shall endeavor to present to you concepts relevant to your immediate needs. I trust I shall find some understanding perceptors.

ELECTRICITY DEFINED RELATIVE TO MIND

I will tell you in advance, for those of you who will poo poo my information for I shall not, nor could I, separate what you call "physical and provable scientific method" from that prana resource which is "mind" and higher dimension. It will only be man in higher dimensional thought who will unravel these puzzles and be able to manifest the physical concept into apparatus.

ELECTRICITY IS THE STRAIN OR TENSION SET UP BY THE TWO OPPOSING DESIRES OF UNIVERSAL MIND THINKING: THE DESIRE FOR BALANCED ACTION AND THE DESIRE FOR REST.

This *electric universe* is a complexity of strains caused by the interaction of these two opposing, interchanging electric desires. All matter is electric. Therefore, all matter is conditioned into greater or lesser strains according to the intensity of desire which is the cause of all electric strain to which it is subjected.

The farther removed from rest the greater the strain or tension. That which we call high electric potential is merely great strain to maintain a condition which is far from the condition of rest.

Now, what might have this to do with viruses which have moved into body cells and won't go away but continue to mutate and violate the central cellular master system? Simple, you pass the proper tonal light frequency through the cells and place such strain on the viruses that they cannot remain "whole" and will diffuse in order to move in the direction of rest. When this has been accomplished the particles again find that rest and when this happens, the strain and tension have been voided. The tension has not BECOME rest, it has simply ceased to be.

The entire electric universe is a complex maze of similar tensions--from the greatest to the smallest. Every particle of matter is separated from its condition of oneness, and each is connected with the other by an electric thread of light which measures the tension of that separateness. Therefore it is obvious that ALL is actually only ONE. Each structure within its societal structure striving for its unity as an operating whole.

I like the example of sodium chloride. When sodium and chlorine desire separateness from their oneness of condition in sodium chloride, an electric strain is set up between that separated Trinity. When the desire for separateness has gone out of sodium and chlorine, the electric tensions which bound them to the rest condition from which they sprang are voided. Likewise sodium and chlorine are utterly voided.

The reason for this is that all matter is a series of electric tensions. When the tensions cease, the conditions set up by them ceases. Here is a most important notation: Electrical tensions exist ONLY between UNBALANCED electrical matter in motion which is separated from other electrical matter in motion. Wherever there is a condition of rest, electricity ceases to be. Electricity is, therefore, a dual force which seemingly unbalances a condition of rest by dividing it into two opposite conditions and setting them in seeming motion. Interchange between the two opposites of motion voids the unbalanced condition at the end of each cycle of electric expression. Therefore, for each cycle there must be the projection and the reflection--to be successful you cannot have half a whole.

Let us consider the apparatus for producing specific strain on an intracellular virus. Well, already you know that you have two very differing entities of differing composition.

MAN AND MATTER EXPRESSED IN CYCLES

You must visualize to understand the cycle of any thing or organism. Take man, for you must think of "generating man" as infant, child and youth. Following his generating cycles come the degenerative ones in which he gradually repays all of his borrowings from his zero of rest and returns to that zero to again borrow power to express the idea of man, etc. This process of Nature, which expresses its cycles of idea in nine lesser cycles, is conspicuously present in the life-death cycles of the elements of matter. Carbon alone expresses the idea of matter. All the nine octaves and major frequencies of the elements are stages of unfoldment and refoldment of carbon. The first four and a half octaves lead to the maturity of carbon by the genero-active contraction of gravity (which is cycled electricity). It is the hardest of all of the other stages of its transition, having the highest melting point (here, once again, you have integration of vibration frequency interrelated with temperature created by that vibration on a given substance). The last four and a half octaves lead from maturity through old age to disappearance at the end of the nine octave cycle by the radioactive expansion of vacuity.

Now, if you would consider the body whole, you would see that if you could maintain the frequency within the master cellular control system, say at the level of maturity you would not need reverse into the degenerative factor.

Now here is another fundamental basic point from which to extend hypotheses. Genero-activity begins at the birth of carbon in the first octave with genero-active, inner explosive speed of light, which is 186,400 miles per second. *It ends with an equal radioactive, outer explosive speed. This speed is the limit at which motion can reproduce itself in curved wave fields before reaching zero where motion and curvature cease.*

CARBON, AMPLITUDE AND OCTAVES

Carbon fulfills the plan of the Creator in His desire to create but one form: the cube-sphere. Carbon alone crystallizes in true cube, with all of the qualities of the true cube and sphere fully exemplified. *All other elements which crystallize as cubes are octave extensions of carbon.* All such extensions occupy the four-zero-four position of wave amplitude.

In carbon are all of the elements of its previous stages, just as in man are all of the actions and reactions of his previous stages. Hydrogen is a one octave younger prototype of carbon. It forms on the wave amplitude at four-zero-four just as carbon forms at four-zero-four one octave ahead. In hydrogen is a whole octave of elemental tones. Several of these have been recently discovered and wrongly labeled isotopes. Isotopes are split tones such as those which a violinist could produce between full tones.

A most amazing thing happens at this point in the unfolding of carbon's life record. Hydrogen's melting point is 259 degrees below zero centigrade and in one octave the winding up process of nature acts like a whiplash at its halfway position where genero-activity and radioactivity meet as equals. This effect tightens the winding of carbon into such a dense substance that the melting point jumps to 3600 degrees above zero in that one octave.

Nature immediately counterbalances this accelerative action by dropping nitrogen, the next element beyond carbon, into a gas which melts at 210 degrees below zero centigrade. It does not recover from the gaseous condition during the rest of its octave.

NEON

Another important note to make is herein. The cosmic seed of the silicon octave is neon.

Nature records every action and desire of the body, likewise every conscious desire and thought of the soul in those cosmic elements which are called "the inert gases"; helium, neon, krypton, argon and some others. These cosmic elements, which will not unite with the physical elements, are the basis of God's recording system by means of which every thought and action of every creating thing is stored in them as seed-extensions from sun and earth centers for repetition until their purposes are fulfilled.

Everything in Nature is purposeful and nothing in Nature fulfills its purpose in one life cycle.

Nature multiplies the time dimensions of her light waves so that patterned records of forms which have expanded beyond man's range of sensing can come within that range, then *divides those time dimensions* until they again disappear into the other half of their cycle beyond man's range of sensing.

When carbon becomes one octave older at the four-zero-four position of cobalt in the sixth octave, it divides its full tone into ten split isotope tones; five on either side.

Carbon has lost much of its vitality and changes its character by thus dividing it into cobalt isotopes. Its melting point has dropped to 1480 degrees, which is slightly higher than the silicon stage of carbon. Because of sharing that position with ten others (isotopes) it has lost much of its true cube-sphere quality of balance which the four-zero-four position manifests. It does, however, become obvious that if an unbalanced particle enters into a previously balanced, let us say, cell and vibrates at a higher dimensional tone it will cause immense strain on the cellular system causing immediate deterioration of the cellular system; now, add to that a substance, say a retrovirus which has the capability of interjecting itself into the very DNA structure, you have an effort at regaining balance--unfortunately to the detriment of the living tissue culture for the carbon creation cannot function and survive in the presence of the attacker.

METALLIC OPPOSITES

I will pass this rather quickly but there will be ones of you who can recognize the importance of these opposing elements. Keep in mind, please, what I just said: "When carbon becomes one octave older at the four-zero-four position of cobalt in the sixth octave, it divides its full tone into ten split isotope tones; five on either side." Let us, however, consider further, the four-zero-four position.

This position is one of balance between pairs of metallic opposites such as iron and nickel, manganese and copper, chromium and zinc or sodium and chloride. When any of these pairs lose their metallic quality, such as iron and oxygen in iron rust, or sodium and chlorine in sodium-chloride, they find both rest and balance in the stony quality of the salts; they crystallize in the cubic system if they are equal or near equal opposite pairs. Sodium-chloride is an excellent example. One can see its approximately true cubes in sodium-chloride (ordinary table salt) or the more distorted cube crystals of sodium-iodide.

The four-zero-four position in the octaves of the elements is the position of rest where any action must end its half cycle and begin its other half. It comes to a point of rest before returning to a point of rest, as all actions and reactions in nature do.

Now, consider a retrovirus which is a crystalline living organism. Specifically recombinant retroviruses--do you see that, in the end, they must recombine to survive for they are basically introduced into alien culture and must adapt their environment to one habitable to their existence?

RHODIUM IN DISINTEGRATION

At one octave of further aging carbon becomes rhodium and again climbs to its amplitude position at four-zero-four by five efforts and descends by five more. Rhodium is more vital than cobalt, for its melting point is 1950 degrees.

The cosmic seed of the rhodium octave is krypton. Great vitality is often evidenceD in nature's creations after they have fully matured. The radioactive death principle is as vital in disintegrating the body as the genero-active principle is in integrating it. That vitality is enhanced by the opposition of the genero-active resistance set up against it. Such strong, vital metals as silver, nickel, copper, tantalum, tungsten, osmium, platinum and gold belong to the next two aging half cycles of carbon.

The next octave of carbon is lutecium and the cosmic seed is xenon. The cosmic seed of carbon's last octave of disappearance arises from the unknown inert gas niton.

OCTAVES UNFOLD FROM THEIR PAST RECORDED SEED AND THEY MUST HAVE A SEED INTO WHICH THEIR PRESENT RECORD CAN REFOLD. THAT PRINCIPLE IS "ABSOLUTE" IN NATURE!

CONSIDER THE INERT GASES

The octaves of the elements of matter "grow" from seed, just as all things grow from seed. From the moment the elements unfold from their seed they are in a constant state of transition, from the beginning of their cycle to the end.

ELEMENTS ARE NOT FIXED CREATED THINGS. THEY ARE PRESSURE CONDITIONS OF LIGHT WAVES.

THOSE CONDITIONS OF LIGHT PRESSURES ARE CONSTANTLY CHANGING FROM INFANCY TO OLD AGE IN THE ELEMENTS OF MATTER JUST AS THEY ARE IN THE ANIMAL KINGDOM. THE

INERT GASES ARE COSMIC ELEMENTS WHICH WILL NOT COMBINE WITH ANY OTHER ELEMENTS.

They constitute the recording system of this creating universe. They surround the zero from which motion springs and to which it returns. They represent minimum motion in the wave, just as amplitudes represent maximum motion. They are the seeds of the octaves of matter, and each octave has a different seed just as different trees have different seeds. Further, they each have a color tone of light ray which is in infinite hues but always of the same "tone" and each has a harmonic frequency which will match its counterpart in matter.

This is why, in dealing with carbon--which man is, you will need to function within the general spectrum of neon which is the seed.

Elements are waves, and waves disappear and reappear. God's recording system does not allow any creating thing to disappear without recording the actions and reactions of its stages of appearance. All states of motion are recorded in the inert gases. In the inert gases are the souls of their bodily manifestations in the universe of motion. In them is desire for expression and the patterned form of that octave.

The cosmic inert gases fill all space between the stars of the heavens. They insulate states of motion from each other by their balancing zero. They bring all motion into being through the will of the Creator, true to the pattern of desire.

There are nine cosmic gases; the first and the last being one. Alphanon begins the cycle and omeganon ends it--to begin again at alphanon. There is no beginning and no ending--just as with soul life. The list of cosmic gases follows: alphanon, betanon, gammanon, helium, neon, argon, krypton, Xenon, niton and omeganon. The ones known to you at this time are helium, neon, argon, krypton and zenon. It is well time for you to be looking beyond.

Dharma, I note this is most tiring and you had several hours of writing for Commander Hatonn prior to our meeting. I would assume the Commander would allow sharing of that early morning document, for you will never again separate man and God and the cycles closing in this particular time of history upon your planet. It will give confirmation that you are not alone for the Lord will send his hosts from the heavens to abide with you, and it has begun in its last countdown. I am most grateful to be chosen for input in these troubled times for my life-stream has been directed, as has yours, to the days of confusion and tribulation. I am most pleased and humble to be included.

I will withdraw that you might take respite. I will be available at your summons.

Thank you for your willing participation and patience with my dawdling. I tend to desire comprehensive information of the subject and we have not the time nor need of such for my work is available for those who can abide the confusion.

I would request another session this day for I wish to analyze the spectrum, for light is the universal language and man has not realized it fully. I consider it most interesting.

Walter Russell to withdraw.

CHAPTER 15

REC. #2 RUSSELL

THURSDAY, OCTOBER 19, 1989 6:15 A.M. YEAR 3, DAY 064

Walter (Russell) present to discuss the matter of the spectrum and do some analytical elaboration. I see that we are moving ahead of the group having to rearrange my punctuation and respell our incorrect printing. I will make an effort to assist a bit more carefully. Your life is so overfilled with duties that I feel most uncomfortable inserting myself to such great extent. I think ones around you do not understand how exhaustive this work becomes.

SPECTRUM ANALYSIS

Light is the universal language. Through spectrum analysis of light waves man has been able to analyze and recognize each element when in its incandescent stage. By means of the spectroscope, you have been enabled to divide light rays through prisms into the component parts which make up the life history of each stage of its two-way cycle.

My colleague, Royal, utilized circular, wedge-shaped, block-crystal quartz prisms to polarize the light to be sent through his scope. You must have the ability to send *every* portion of the spectrum through the prism. That portion is selectable, so that a very narrow band corresponding to any color from infra-red up through the visible colors and then through the entire ultra-violet range -- in extremely narrow steps, can be selected for use in illuminating the specimens. As you encounter mutants of a given frequency of a particle, bacteria, virus, etc., you will find very, very critical and minute variations of perfect attunement. However, do not let this mislead you for remember, the perfection of attunement must be with the perfect cell so that stress is maintained on the invader particle.

Your problem becomes significant in that destruction comes rapidly, even in a most slowly growing retrovirus, in the integration with the DNA structure. The most desirable time for correction is, of course, before that invasion takes place.

This is where "preventive medicine", if you will, will be your method of choice--in other words, once perfected and your frequencies pretty well assumed, you will treat the "well" body on a rather regular basis.

You will find such increased well-being, prolonged perfection and renewal of the whole body that it will be a most sought-after therapy, or ongoing treatment, for a healthy society.

Each and every element tells the story of its entire previous "incarnations" in other octaves, since its beginning. Any line in one octave is repeated in the next, but shifted in position because of the changing pressures of each succeeding octave. Let us use hydrogen for discussion.

The spectrum of hydrogen is preponderantly red. A bright red line indicates its present octave. Other red lines tell its past history in lower octaves.

Let us say that you take the history of hydrogen, as compared to the complex spectrum of say, iron and it becomes like the history of an obscure child as compared to that of Alexander the Great.

In the spectrum analysis of iron, for instance, the lines which belong to iron and those which tell its recent and remote history can be seen at a glance. These lines also indicate the relative ability of the iron atom to charge or discharge. Wave length 7181.8 is *immediately* recognizable as belonging to iron in its present octave; 6916.8 is recent history and 6944.8 is extremely remote history, and so forth.

The visible and invisible spectrum is divided into several thousand lines. Each line is different in its shade of color and in its plane. Each line proves that this universe of varying motion is a universe of varying pressures. When the color is invisible it still carries a very specific frequency.

There is a number which will correlate in all instances to all work. It may be a square-of, a sum-of, a division-of, a multiple-of, etc., etc., of a harmonic of a given "thing":

THAT NUMBER IS 169443 WHICH IN TURN IS EQUAL TO THE HARMONICS OF MASS AT THE CENTER OF A LIGHT FIELD. IT IS ALSO ASSOCIATED WITH STRUCTURE OF THE ATOM.

HETERODYNING LIGHT

Let us consider an observed fact in physics. This is a principle used in radio and in work with sound. When two different frequencies of vibration are produced, they inter-act upon each other to produce two new frequencies--one of which is the sum of the two original or fundamental frequencies, the other is the difference between the two originating or fundamental frequencies. As a good example in the range of sound; take, say, a tone of 400 cycles per second and another tone of 600 cycles per second, the resulting new frequencies will then be 200 cycles per second--or the difference, and 1,000 cycles for the other *new* tone, the sum.

Royal applied this principle to the field of light. The visible frequencies range from about 436 trillion oscillations per second at the red end of the visible spectrum, to about 732 trillion oscillations per second at the violet end of the visible spectrum. An oscillatory rate faster than 732 trillion times per second results in a beam which is in the invisible, ultra-violet range. The ultra-violet band occupies several octaves of vibration, as compared to the visible spectrum which occupies less than one octave of vibration. *The upper limit of an octave has twice the vibratory rate of the lower limit of the same octave.*

Therefore, the range of the vibratory light spectrum invisible to the human eye is larger than the frequency range of the light spectrum which the human eye can perceive and for your current endeavors, you will be working most diligently in your blind range for the most part.

You accomplish the process of this light by bringing an invisible, ultra-violet beam of, say, 1,200 trillion oscillations per second into contact with another equally-invisible beam of say, 1,700 trillion oscillations per second; the difference between the oscillatory rates of the two originating beams results in the production of a light beam having an oscillatory rate of 500 trillions per second, which is within the range visible to the human eye.

Oh yes, Dharma, there are ones about your place who *almost* understand this. Actually, they understand this quite well, it is just that there are the missing links in all puzzles. We will give you some researchers who are outstanding in their progressive work at the end of this document. We will not do so now, for segments of this paper are going forth and a thing out of its time is almost sure to perish at the hands of the indiscreet.

Many micro-organisms could only be observed, in the past, if stained with a chemical. Some micro-organisms never became visible with other microscopes, because no suitable stain could be found. What is more important is that with the addition of stains, the frequencies are altered and correct readings cannot be determined. Royal's microscope had the prime advantage in that he could locate many micro-organisms having no color in the visible light range--their frequency characteristic is such that they have a "color" in the invisible, ultra-violet range. By the use of the heterodyning principle in his microscopes as mentioned, the micro-organisms of ultra-violet colors are brought into the visible light range in their natural state, without the use of any stain. Because of the breakdown of the cycling assumption, you will also find that much is similar in the infra-red scope. The heterodyning principle in the scope also brings into visibility the micro-organisms which had not responded to any known stain, and all micro-organisms can be viewed in their natural state. This gives the investigator a considerable advantage for in addition to a stain changing the frequency it has another great disadvantage--it kills the organism.

This is the only method, further, which allows viewing of organisms in their living state--ELECTRON MICROSCOPES INSTANTLY KILL ANY LIVING ORGANISMS WITH THE BEAMS PROJECTED.

Further, consider this, which is most often overlooked. As you attune frequency, you are not "just" bringing the invisible into visible--*BUT YOU ARE ALSO CAUSING THE CLUTTER OF THE VISIBLE TO BECOME INVISIBLE---NOT A LOT DIFFERENT FROM VIEWING A SO-CALLED UFO, EXCEPT THAT THE UFO WILL BRING ITS FREQUENCY TO MATCH THE VIEWER AND THE VIEWER, THEREFORE, DOES NOT LOSE HIS ENVIRONMENTAL PERCEPTION.* This is another area, the UFO phenomenon of visibility, which is greatly connected to 169443--a very important numerical arrangement indeed.

CONSIDER ATOMIC STRUCTURE

Elements of matter are not different substances, or different "things". They are different pressure conditions of light waves. The light units of the elements are all alike but are differently conditioned by the electric pressures exerted upon them during the inward or outward spiral journey from zero to zero.

The unanswered mystery of how the elements become mathematically precise octave tones, just as musical tones or color tones of the spectrum are mathematically precise in vibration orderliness, lies in the wave field gyroscope principle.

Together the eight elements of an octave form two halves of one whole cycle of tones which ascend from zero to the four-zero position of amplitude and descend again to zero to begin again. This spiral journey contracts into greater pressures as it approaches wave field amplitude positions at spiral apices, and expands into lower ones on the return journey to spiral bases.

Location of elements on wave fields are determined by wave-field mirrors. The two-way spiral journey of each *half* cycle extends between six mirrors of still light which compose the wave-field, and winds around a still shaft which centers the spiral. Three of these mirrors are the mirrors of action and, of course, the other three are the mirrors of reaction. The three of action are the inner intersection planes of the cube and the three of reaction are the outer boundary planes of the wave field.

All of these planes of the wave field are of zero curvature but, the spiral universe which is forming within those planes is curved. Curved planes of light act as two-way lenses which bend light to focal points and extend it from those focal points radially.

As the two-way spirals of forming matter extend from the wave field center in opposite directions toward wave field intersections, the six mirror planes of still light focus three points of still light upon the still shaft of each half cycle. Centers are formed at these focal points which become the one, two, three positive and negative elements of matter by rotating gyroscopically upon the wheels of light which act as equators for those borning tones.

Multiplying and dividing pressures determine the density and volume of each succeeding element. *The color spectrum records these pressures, as the complete history of every element, from octave to octave of the whole nine octave cycle of the elements.*

Keep in mind, that multiplying pressures of the spiral also affect the curvature of its light lenses to such an extent that the focusing positions change their mathematical ratios in conformity with the acceleration of gravity and the deceleration of radiation.

GYROSCOPIC PRINCIPLE

The positions of focal centers of gyroscopic wheels, in the gyroscopic principle, are thusly affected; each element is the square of the distance to and from its succeeding one, in accordance with its direction. The direction of gravity is the inverse square, and the opposite direction is the direct square. The volume of each succeeding element is likewise affected directly and inversely as the cube.

Six of the eight gyroscopic wheels of the whole octave are thus accounted for by geometric projection of two-way opposed lights through each other, from two sets of three mirror boundary fields. The fourth double tone is formed at the rest point where eight cube wave fields meet. This is the point of rest which is known as the center of gravity in earths or suns---where motion and curvature cease.

The completed sphere thus becomes a section of eight adjoining wave fields and revolves around that point of rest upon the wave shaft where the two half cycles of the wave meet. For this reason the four-zero-four position is one of balance in which the yellow of orange is the dominating color of one of its two gyroscopic wheels and the yellow of green is the other, centered, of course, by "white".

At the two points upon the still shaft of the turning sphere where the shaft penetrates its surface are the magnetic poles of still light which control the balance of each sphere's turning. One of these is the north magnetic pole which controls the winding of the sphere into density by centripetal electric force, and the other is the south magnetic pole which controls its unwinding into space.

In a sphere such as our nearly mature sun, these magnetic poles are practically upon the sun's pole of rotation, but upon oblating planets, such as your earth, the magnetic poles are removed from that pole of rotation in accordance with the measure of the earth's oblateness.

The elements of matter are miniature stellar systems. Every principle and law which applies to one applies to the other. This solar system is a gyroscopic wheel in the position which iron occupies in the elemental series. When it spirals a little further it will correspond to a carbon atom. At that occurrence the sun will then be a true sphere and its new planets will also be true spheres. Now, isn't this a most fascinating and wondrous journey into revelation? I realize it appears most complex but the principles are most simple indeed.

The gyroscopic principle accounts for the law of Nature which causes like elements to seek one another. All decomposing compounds are sorted out, element by element, gyroscopically.

The efforts of man to transmute one element into another must be governed by this principle, and not upon the theory that another substance will be obtained by "knocking out an electron". It makes no difference how many planets there are in a solar or atomic system in so far as its "substance" as an element is concerned. One or more added or subtracted would not change the element into another substance any more than one or more children would affect the nationality of the parents.

Transmutation will become simplified by observing that the plane of gyration, in relation to amplitude, and the speed of revolution of the gyroscopic wheel upon its still shaft, will alone change volume by either multiplying or dividing density. Great possibilities in new metals lie in the proper application of this principle.

This, of course, is where our Master St. Germain is most adept; in the fields of alchemy and transmutation--therefore, you can surmise that you will find the solutions to many of the mysteries solved in the violet ray spectrum--but that is another story for another day.

Dharma, it has been a most long and tedious session. Please let us take a break and then we will resume with a discussion about the "shape" of the universe--not the social status but rather that it is in no shape at all. Thank you for you extended attention for which my appreciation is unlimited.

I will herewith withdraw my presence that you might take respite.
Most cordially,

Walter Russell

CHAPTER 16

REC. #3, RUSSELL

THURSDAY, OCTOBER 19, 1989 12:45 P.M. YEAR 3, DAY 064

Walter to continue.

SHAPE OF THE UNIVERSE

In this instance, it might appear that the shape of the universe would have very little to do with our subject matter; however, it is most relative.

The fact is, that this infinite and ageless universe HAS NO SHAPE. It has a seeming infinite extension, but that extension is a reflected one. This is a most important fact for it can explain many things and misperceptions of things such as time and space. This electric universe of two-way extended light is but a series of mirrors which reflect into each other through curved lenses. Its seeming extension might be likened to a light within a mirror-bounded room. One light within such a mirrored enclosure would seemingly extend infinitely, but the light thus mirrored would be the same light. The reflected extension would have, actually, no reality whatsoever.

The idea of continuity or discontinuity is based upon mirrored effect of an initial cause. Continuity infers "time". Time is but one of the effects which constitutes this universe. Time flows two separate ways, but the senses detect only the forward flow. They cannot detect the backward flow which cancels out the forward flow. Time is as unreal as the wave universe is unreal.

What is true in principle of one wave is true of all waves. Each wave is a two-way reflected extension of an equilibrium zero which we call a vibration. Vibrations appear, disappear and reappear from their source of rest to manifest an idea which is existent alone in rest. Just as the vibration of one wave disappears into its zero of universal stillness, so do all vibrations disappear into the universal zero of stillness. This zero universe of vibrating waves can have no shape other than a seeming one.

THE PRINCIPLE OF VOIDING

This is a zero universe of seeming mechanical motion of force exerted in a seeming three-dimensional universe.
Every action of any nature begins with zero, counts up to nine, to end and begin again at zero. Beyond nine it cannot go, but up to nine it must go. Nine is universal. It is universal because it is the wave field number--the eight of the cube centered by the zero of gravity in the sphere.

Consider your decimal system, it is based upon the wave field of the cube sphere, and is as follows:

0-1-2-3-4-0-4-3-2-1-0
equals 10-1-2-3-4-5-6-7-8-9-10

The musical scale and the spectrum of Nature correspond to the wave field tones. They are as follows:

musical 0 - 1 - 2 - 3 - 4 - 3 - 2 - 1 - 0
tones do - re - mi - fa - sol - fa - mi - re - do
(Keynote) (Overtone) (Keynote)

spectrum:
black red red-orange yellow white yellow green blue black
tones:
violet violet

The planes are centered by zero. All intersections of these planes add up to eight. Eight, centered by their zero source, equals nine. Likewise the cube itself adds up to eight by counting the intersections of its six faces. Further, there are eight directions of action and eight of reaction; each eight being four pairs, which are nine by adding the centering zero.

Dharma, I believe it would be most helpful to have a drawing at this point. Is there some way to allow space within the writing?

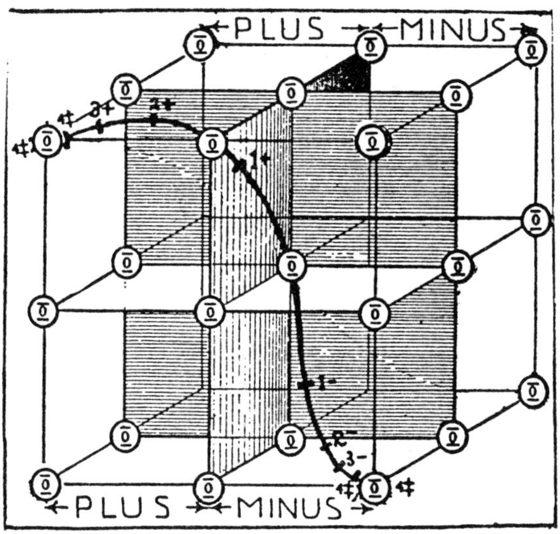

Locations of elements on wave fields are determined by wave-field mirrors

Thank you. I find that I work greatly with illustrations but we will not concern with that at present for most of my scratchings are available.

Nine is the three times three of length, breadth and height extended from zero. The length, breadth and heigth of any expression is two extended zeros centered by zero. Length and breadth are static, for they are both on equipotential levels. Height is dynamic, for it is radial.

The universal nine of matter and space is three mirrors of rest, centered by rest, from which all three extend at right angles to each other, each mirroring itself into the other.

The universal nine of the octave is four pairs of opposite pressures extending diagonally from zero which centers the cube to eight zeros which corner the cube.

The measure of extension from zero to zero is desire for extension. Desire for extension from zero to zero is energy in zero. Energy extended from zero to zero is manifested by pressures of desire equally multiplied and divided--equally added and subtracted--equally credited and debited--and equally and oppositely conditioned. The sum of all these balanced effects is zero.

Zero pressures equally multiplied and divided are manifested by the action and reaction of motion. Motion is a projection of the opposed energy pressures of desire from within a centering zero to the extended mirrors of rest, which measure desire and mirror it back to rest in the centering zero as expressed desire. The sum of dually reflected motion thus expressed is zero. Please understand that I do not use the term "desire" as the usually careless term of lustful eroticism.

Zero thus extended by action to fulfill desire for expression, and simultaneously mirrored back to manifest the fulfillment of expressed desire, is all there is to this universe of rest. Zero multiplied or divided--added or subtracted--extended or retracted--results in zero. This is a zero universe in all effects of motion--a seeming universe in time and sequence--and a mirage universe of imagined form.

It is a universe of two negations which simultaneously cancel each other and sequentially repeat the cancelling of their negations to create the illusion that zero can be multiplied--or divided--or added to--or subtracted from--to create a reality which never is nor can become.

That is what creation is. It is the imagining of knowing. Knowing is Light. Light is still. Imagining is thinking. Thinking is the imagined action and reaction of motion mirrored from zero of rest to zero of rest.

<u>This is a still universe of the Light of knowing. In it is no activity</u>.

We would request that your son, Paul, be given great credit for his arrival at the understanding of this theory in what he called Dimensional Life. Please also understand, Dharma, that to be thrust into this kind of information at twenty-five years of age in a tormented and ridiculing world could never have produced the attention it both deserved and merited. What appeared as a senseless waste in death (and dear one, it was not suicide) was in actuality the only way this information could be funneled and utilized for mankind. It was careless planning on the part of the evil enemy but as the events occurred, you took the load and we can bring it forth in spite of the loss. At Paul's age and the medical perception of mental illness, he would have been incarcerated for insanity and the material would have been lost. This is given in an effort to unfold some of the great and painful puzzles of your life journey.

You must hold in your heart, as the hours of fatigue fall upon you and the body waivers; as the intent is softened by the continuous bombarding and actual jeopardy of life itself, that these are the ending and beginning of times and we are about the saving of a species of man from extinction. I know you cannot comprehend this for you and your ones are most humble and selfless; but your rewards for this service shall be without limits. There are ones upon your place who consider themselves to have all the answers and they in turn, push aside truth in the young ones who all but wallow in the path of their feet. It is most sad indeed.

Well, you ones say, all this about illusion and no motion cannot be truth for your senses tell you otherwise. Your senses are most inadequate. They deceive you mightily. That, however, is so, else the play of Creation could not be played. The senses record but little of the whole. If the senses could but see the whole there would be no play. The senses record motion alone for the senses themselves are but motion. Motion is an illusion which only *seems* to be. It has no being.

The senses do not <u>know</u>, but man believes that his senses do <u>know</u> and in that belief lies man's confusion.

The senses, being but motion, sense moving things, and moving light mirrored as moving things. They sense the forward movement of an airplane piling up compression ahead of it--but they do not record the mirrored invisible counterpart of that plane--equal to it in potential and speed--moving backward into a vacuum behind the plane which simultaneously voids the compression ahead of it. The inadequacy of the senses to record the backward flow of forward moving things--causes the illusions of sequence and time. In this principle, every element in the whole known series, is simultaneously intergrated and balanced by disintegration. No time interval elapses between the debiting of any credit extended to opposites in Nature.

Dharma, could we have one more sketch, please.

THIS UNIVERSE OF MATTER IS COMPOSED OF PAIRS OF NEGATIONS WHICH NEVER EXCEED ZERO

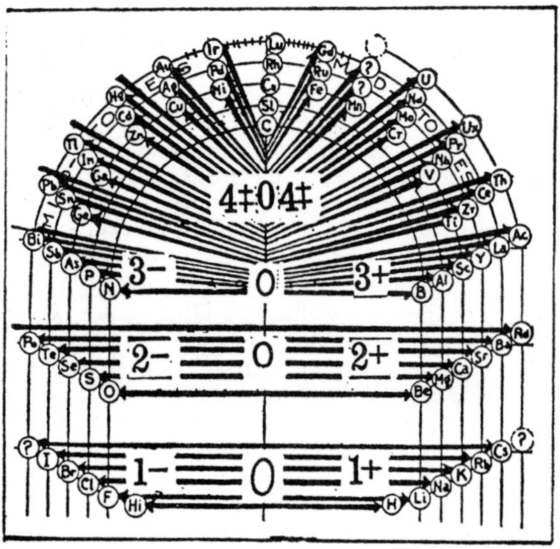

Each one of these elemental pairs are equal and opposite mirrored extensions from a centering zero fulcrum. I believe we mentioned early on in this document that we would, among other things be proving the presence, or existence, of God. Well, the fulcrum of all effect is the One Light of God. Pure and total ALL INCLUSIVE.

GOD ALONE IS--IN MAN--AND IN ALL THINGS

For one man, known in his last earth journey as Walter Russell, was given these things in the same manner as you are being given these things. My proof did not confront me until I transitioned where I now live in the midst of that truth. I am most grateful and blessed to have this opportunity of working in retrospect for so few have the opportunity.

I trust I have given you sufficient data to allow conclusions that if you are to survive the current plague upon mankind you must act quickly and you must remove yourselves from orthodox hogwash. The microscope and apparatus of Royal Rife is mandatory to your success. Through its use you can discover the frequency characteristics of micro-organisms, you can observe micro-organisms not shown by other microscopes, you can ascertain information regarding the relationship between mirco-organisms and their chemical environment and then, the prize---you can use selected frequencies of radiation to destroy specific micro-organisms.

I further would like to suggest that ones work closely with John F. Crane and his associate, Mark L. Gallert. Further, much refraction and frequency information will come forth from one John Schroepfer in conjunction with the circle of researchers which must be pulled together into a working unit. Each will have a contribution for it is not to be that only one entity shall carry the whole but rather it must come forth from multiple carriers of specific portions. This is the only method of security for the devices and the human workers.

It is further mandatory that ones who are given assistance for their contribution by interim medications and substances, through these channels, be dedicated to the funding and development of the cure for AIDS. This IS the cure and anything short of a cure is totally inadequate. The quality of life can be improved and length of life extended but there is presently no "medical" cure for these retrovirus induced death diseases. Further, if there would be such it would never pass the protocol examination and be made available to the public in a timely manner.

This data will get mammoth audience and demand for interim products will be tremendous. We will not place that information into the public unless we have dedicated commitment from those in the development of such a product. Currently there is such a product to which Commander Hatonn has previously made reference. This product is not yet marketed but shows great promise. The time of the lie is past; man must have truth and he must be given a means of curing his plight--it is already too late for many dear ones.

I will take the liberty herein to quote a dissertation by my collegue, John Crane. I honor him by so-doing, further, it is most difficult to get his attention from these etheral dimensions in order to obtain permission.

ELECTRON THERAPY --- John F. Crane

"Eradication of disease is the exciting promise of new discoveries in microscopy and radio wave electron transfer by Royal R. Rife.

"Virus diseases, the ancient scourge of man, which still plague millions in the world, are destroyed by modulated radio waves, tuned to precise frequencies in thousands of lab tests. The frequency instruments have killed organisms in test tubes, animals, and human patients. The lethal rays are transmitted by the frequency instrument ray tubes. Most cases respond within a period of two months and diseases are quickly rendered non-infectious. Destruction of the organisms by rays is described as being similar to the phenomenon of transmitted electron energy and coordinating resonance of critical frequencies with electromagnetic and static fields.

"Rife has demonstrated that the frequency instruments have the power to kill germs without harm to human tissue.

"Development of the ray to the point where it is now used effectively against virus, bacteria and fungi has been accomplished and made possible by two other discoveries of nearly equal importance to practitioners and lab workers. One has been the design and construction by Rife of powerful virus microscopes, with special illumination and peak magnification beyond 17,000x. The other is Rife's isolation of pure cultures of the filterable forms of virus, which are too small to be seen with the best research microscopes. Virus has been revealed for the first time as the prenatal cell of pathogenic disease and is viewed by the heterodyne wave length of light transmitted through the virus."

Now, I shall positively disintegrate Dharma's day and cause her to sign off--in love I trust. I have Royal Rife here at my side so I only take liberty with Mr. Crane, not Royal. I felt I should leave you with just a bit of humor. I am given commitment that he will not impose his presence upon your kind mind. If you ones pool your resources, you have all of that which you need to successfully bring this project to positive fruition.

I most surely add emphasis to the request of Commanders Hatonn and Ashtar---get the research facility away from the coastal area of the Pacific. Bring it to the higher ground of this mountain village. I will not divulge locations but it is most imperative that the work not be lost to earthquake or other disasters.

Perhaps ones could combine efforts and present a cost estimate for laboratory items and full time researchers who would require travel expenses, etc. It is apparent to me that the public should make immediate contribution to such a cause. If ones can write a check for AIDS research as did Mr. Forbes, perhaps he could contribute to the cure and not just the ongoing comfort of the disease. Those who are not of the elite "controllers" must take a stand in defense of you wondrous people of the lie--this is about the extinction of your species and it is not equitable that a few keep it from the masses.

I shall withdraw for this session, Dharma. I thank you for your most necessary capabilities. Our intent is to not bury ones in confusing information but we desire to keep contact to a minimum for your safety. Please understand that our overall vision far surpasses yours of that plane and we must act wisely and with caution of you ones. You ones must take equal care and security of your brothers.

I will now take my leave, in love and appreciation,

Walter Russell-

CHAPTER 17

REC. #1 HATONN

FRIDAY, OCTOBER 20, 1989 7:00 A.M. YEAR 3, DAY 065

Hatonn present to respond to inquiries. However, shortly I shall have to request a relief from personal inquiries for we must get this material of current crises finished and ones forget that Hatonn, Ashtar, etc., utilize the scribe's time in equal measure.

Commander Ashtar acknowledges "Victory's" petition for wholeness of his hip. He does request that you look carefully within to see that which you are doing and desiring. Is the wholeness for the purpose of ego or true need? Ones must be most careful in exuberance that the trap of personal "I shall show the world" ego does not entrap the physical manifestation. Ones must become most selfless for the purposes of the dark brotherhood are served more readily than are the purposes of God. Victory, you must carefully consider actions and intent and personal responsibility rather than press-ahead, no-matter-what to cause public uproar and attention.

The ones in this locale need secrecy and no attention whatsoever. Be most cautious, son, in your passion or you will fall of that passion misused. Other actions of responsibility and selflessness speak more loudly than a loud, cacophony of "a spectacle". We need no more "spectacles"; we need dedicated, "melt-in" workers who call no enemy attention unto our camp. This particular encampment from whence comes these documents is most critical indeed and at this time, must have NO ATTENTION WHATSOEVER! Too much display of passion will cause ones to be locked-away in the name of fanaticism and sometimes, rightfully so. We must not have attention drawn to this placement for, as yet, it is still most premature. Please, no one take personal offense to these writings for lessons must go forth unto all; we have not time for personal detail so ones who receive must look within for intent. We do not come forth to reprimand in hardly any instance and when we do so--WE REALLY DO SO AND TELL YOU QUITE BLUNTLY THAT YOU HAVE BLOWN IT. SO BE IT AND PEACE UNTO YOU ALL FOR IT IS THE TIME OF RECOGNIZING YOUR HUMAN-NESS AND RISING ABOVE IT WITH SELF-DISCIPLINE AND TRUTH--NOT LOUD VOICE AND EMPTY WORDS--SPEAK SO THAT THE WORLD LISTENS AND JOINS YOU IN PEACE, NOT ALTERCATION FOR YOUR PERSONAL STANCE. *MAN AS A WHOLE HAS BEEN BETRAYED, NOT JUST THE INDIVIDUALS, AND YOU ONES MUST HOLD THAT MOST CLOSELY IN YOUR HEARTS FOR IN THE ENDING THE "ALL" IS BUT THE "WHOLE OF THE MANY"*.

Let me give you good news. When you think the "public" is attuned and is alert and "after you", look again. It has taken from the 17th to the eve of the 19th for the ones in control of the San Francisco freeway breakdown, to realize there were not as many cars as projected on the freeway due to the ball games, and further, continue to say how much worse it might have been with all those people stuffed into that stadium. Man, in general, is so unaware that he is most apt to overlook that which is directly under his nose and before his eyes.

Be most observant these coming few days--the sun flare cosmic rays will be bombarding you most heavily---IT IS THE TIME, HOWEVER, FOR YOU IN "FREE ENERGY" EXPERIMENTATION INTO COLD FUSION TO MOVE YOUR ASSETS!!

Now, I would most like to respond to J.S. regarding Satan as a being or a force. It is most difficult to respond in any sense relative to perception of human input. Bear with me please as I would have preferred to have Sananda or Germain or Michael respond to this matter, however, Ashtar and myself, have created the question so I will endeavor to respond--as in fourth dimension perception which is not so removed from your status.

I will insert, however, that one of the very next documents will cover the subject of "EVIL" in great substance. It was not originally intended that Dharma would need carry the burden of the myriad of fragmented subject matter, but ones of the scribes who had been intended to share the load, have stumbled into traps along the way. We will do the best we can in the limitations of human "time". Please be kind if our answers are not as full as would be desirable.

Is Satan "real"? I must respond with a question: "Is Christ `real'?" Is the physical format "real"? NO! NOT IN THE PHYSICAL SENSE OF THE QUESTION AS ASKED. YES! IN THE TRUE SENSE OF PERCEPTION OF CONSCIOUSNESS.

I REQUEST THAT THIS PERSONAL ENTRY BE ALLOWED TO REMAIN IN THIS DOCUMENT FOR ON THE YESTER DAY'S WRITING, SIR RUSSELL GAVE YOU A MOST "SCIENTIFIC" PROOF OF THE FACT THAT ALL IS LIGHT, GOD IS THE CENTRAL "WHOLE" LIGHT OF THE ZERO FULCRUM AND ALL IS A REFLECTION OF CONCEPTUAL PERCEPTION--AN ILLUSION, IF YOU WILL.

Now, your senses tell you that you are manifested reality--you are massive thought form and you are stuck with that perception; therefore, the circumstance must be handled through a drastic change of the "CAUSAL POINT", that the reflection and perception be a redirection of the energy flow--since ALL is MIND--the MIND of individual and "whole" must be redirected into truth and away from the incorrect "illusion". NOW, ISN'T THIS JUST THE MOST WONDROUS GAME OF UNIVERSAL INTRIGUE? I DO NOT JEST, THIS IS THE MOST WONDROUS EXPERIENCE ALLOWED FOR THE MIND OF MAN WHO WAS CREATED BY CREATOR, WITHIN THE CREATION, FOR THE SUBSTANCE OF REFLECTED LIGHT-ENERGY FROM THE CREATOR SOURCE, ITSELF, GIVEN THE GIFT OF FREE-WILL CHOICE AND NON-JUDGMENTAL ALLOWANCES OF ACTION---ACTION/MOTION, TOO, IS AN ILLUSION WHICH YOU WILL MOVE BEYOND IN YOUR

TRANSITION INTO HIGHER TRUTH WITHOUT TIME OR SPACE LIMITATIONS. THIS IS NOT ONLY NOT "AGAINST" THE UNIVERSAL LAWS---IT "IS" THE LAW OF THE CREATION AND COSMIC PHYSICS.

MY DEAR FRIENDS, YOU ARE THE REFLECTION OF THE GOD SOURCE EXPERIENCING IN HIS CHOSEN FORMAT--"HIS WONDROUS 'PLAY', IF YOU WILL.

THERE IS NO WAY TO "EXPLAIN" A CONCEPT AS PERSONAL AS THE BREATHING OF AN INDIVIDUAL. YOU WHO WORK SO CLOSELY IN THE NETWORK OF PULLING THESE THOUGHT FRAGMENTS BACK INTO FOCUS AND SPIRALING BACK INTO SOURCE MUST REALIZE HOW WELL YOU ARE TENDED FOR YOU ARE THE CONDUITS FOR THE FOCUSING OF SUCH MAGNIFICENT ENERGY SO THAT THE PLAY CLOSES IN PERFECTION AND THE STAGE BE SET FORTH FOR THE NEXT.

I RUN A RISK AT THIS POINT, IN PRESENTING SUCH A DISCUSSION, FOR WE WILL LOSE, AT THIS POINT, SOME VERY DEDICATED RESEARCHERS---SO BE IT, FOR IF WE DO NOT MOVE IN "TRUTH", THEN WE SHALL NOT MOVE AT ALL; DO I SPEAK CLEARLY? ALLOW IT TO PENETRATE FOR THE SEEMINGLY UNEXPLAINABLE IS THE SIMPLE AND LEAST COMPLEX EXPLANATION OF ALL. WHEN YOU COME INTO UNDERSTANDING, THE METHODS AND ANSWERS POUR FORTH LIKE UNTO A WATERFALL. HOWEVER, THE MASS OF MAN IS STILL SLEEPING AND DREAMING ON THE REFLECTIONS FED UNTO HIM BY ALL SORTS OF COSMIC MIND FRAGMENTS AND TO THIS POINT, REFUSES TO OPEN HIS MIND AND PERCEIVE THAT WHICH IS TRUTH. IT BECOMES THE OLD PRACTICE OF "IF I CLOSE MY EYES IT WILL GO AWAY; IF I REFUSE TO LOOK AND SEE, THEN IT CANNOT BE REAL"! NAY, WE WILL NOT GO AWAY, NOR WILL YOUR "PROBLEMS" SOLVE THEMSELVES; YOU HAVE MANIFESTED THEM AND YOU WILL "CURE" THEM.

The term "fallen angels" is, of course, a misrepresentation but we are stuck with your vocabulary which presents different perceptions to different ones. If we do not speak in terms which the masses understand and can relate unto, we can never reach a point of acceptance of that which is truth--we must begin slowly and work our way through. NO ONE ON YOUR PLACE IS TRULY READY FOR TOTAL UNDERSTANDING OF HOW IT ACTUALLY *IS*! You have had man paint his perceptions in myriads of ways to the point that you can no longer even perceive how it really is------how many truly understood my dissertation on illusion? Be honest--TRULY understand!

Beloved Lucifer is quite 'real'---Satan, as you recognize the energy. In the higher dimensions of perception, there are energies of higher status than the third dimensional state of perception. These ones are guides, tormentors, experience makers----et cetera. Just as there are the wondrous energies of Christ consciousness and guides that work within the lighted perceptions, so, too, are there the dark brotherhood guides and energy forms. These we refer to as "fallen angels" simply because they cling to the Satanic consciousness and "angels" are discarnate energy forms. You ones wish to place your "heaven" somewhere above you--out there somewhere; therefore anything displaced from that realm of experience in human terms, must "fall" down from somewhere--to somewhere. These are simply the energy form guides and "persuaders" of the dark brotherhood of Evil.

There is a most important point to be repeated herein, "Evil" as an energy form most surely exists and it comes from the Satanic forces--the blackest negative void of all action and reaction, and you better consider it very `real' for through these perceived actions and reactions will come the placement of your own energy (soul) form during and at the closing of the play.

Mankind will play out his parts exactly as written, for he has yet no mass perception that it COULD be different. He mouths a lot of words, but man will not change the scenario--just as man will find and present the solution and cure for AIDS, he will not do so until the appropriate number of energies have changed dimensions for he expects it to be so--it is the reflection he accepts.

Then why do we continue to pound and experience? Because we CAN effect change and, unchecked, AIDS can annihilate the species. DO YOU HEAR WHAT I SAY? IT CAN, AND UNCHECKED IT WILL, ANNIHILATE THE SPECIES OF EARTH MAN.

Oh, but you say: "Well, you said that some self-elite ones have the method of cure and will use it. What about them? So the species would not perish. You are nuts, Hatonn." No, I am not nuts, for the evil will be removed and will no longer exist at the end of the play. That means if you add zero to zero you end with zero! You do your own mathematics.

Still a bit confusing and dense? So be it as that conclusion removes the arrogance and allows the truth to be taught unto you.

You will not, as such, walk down the road and meet Mr. Satan and his band of fallen angels---or will you? It is all in consciousness--Christ consciousness or Satanic consciousness, of which will you be the tool? Which "army" are you serving, and to what extent? Do you completely follow the Laws of the Creation or do you fudge just a bit on almost all counts? You see, there is the summit on either side--the deliberate serving of the "Devil" in Satanic ritual practice; or the Cosmic Christ goodness and purity within the Laws of The Creation. In between, lay all the grey areas whereby the self-"judgment" shall fall upon you from time to time---where will you experience next---with the Christ consciousness or the Satanic consciousness? That, brothers, is free-will choice.

This has naught to do with the mystics or mysticism of what you like to refer to as the NEW-AGE MOVEMENT. That path will lead you right into the lion's den, my friends. Just as the erroneous assumption that you will somehow "float up to the clouds and abide there--some way or another". YOU MUST HAVE THE KNOWLEDGE OF TRUTH TO ATTAIN THAT WHICH

YOU CLAIM TO SEEK. BURY YOUR HEAD AND REFUSE TO HEAR WILL NOT MAKE TRUTH DIFFERENT; IT ONLY ASSURES YOU LESS THAN WHAT IS YOURS TO GLEAN FROM THIS EXPERIENCE. EACH MUST OPEN HIS OWN EYES AND STOP PULLING ANOTHER INTO HIS OWN TRAP OF IGNORANCE AND, FURTHER, MUST BE FLEXIBLE ENOUGH TO RECEIVE OF THE INPUT SO THAT THERE IS EVIDENCE FROM WHICH TO MAKE A JUST DECISION.

We come forth in daring disclosure of how it is so that you can find and enforce your own proof of our truth. If it appears as doom and gloom, then I suggest you make an HONEST appraisal of that which is going on around you from within self--depression, stress, unhappiness, etc.--to that which is abounding in your entire world as a whole. You are connected to each and every portion of the whole--YOU cannot break away--if it goes, you all go. Like it or not, you are ultimately stuck within the mire of the whole, you cannot get off this orb--until you change dimensions, with or without physical format, you are STUCK! You have proved that you live in a gross lie--WOULD YOU PLEASE JUST TAKE A LITTLE CHANCE AND TRY US? SO BE IT, MAY YOU BE GIVEN TO RECEIVE OF THE WORD FOR THE TIME IS AT HAND.

Dear John, I hope that I have not just further confused the issue in point but as I check my sensors of our connection, I believe you are content until we can take the matter up more fully.

Our thrust in these journals is to allow you to come into your trust of truth from our source and then we can interchange in open platform that you can come into knowledge. Do not despair too greatly, millions will be lost for they will refuse to accept while they wait and wait and wait for the truth THEY EXPECT! IF YOU ARE AWAITING, IN DETAIL, FOR THAT WHICH MAN SAID GOD SAID, YE SHALL MOST SURELY BE WAITING INTO INFINITY--WHICH, IN MOST INSTANCES, WILL NOT BE OF SUCH PLEASANT EXPERIENCE. PULL UP YOUR HEADS FROM YOUR SANDPILES AND TAKE A LOOK AROUND. IF WE DO NOT BRING TRUTH WHAT HAVE YOU LOST TO HEAR OF US? WE BRING NO FRAGMENT OF EVIL SO IT COULD NOT BE DAMAGING UNTO YOU---WE URGE YOU LOOK AT THE OTHER SIDE--LOOK AT THAT WHICH CLAIMS, OF ITS OWN RIGHT, TO BE EVIL AND THEN KEEPS YOU LOCKED IN IGNORANCE BY IMPOSING LIMITS UPON YOURSELVES.

I TELL YOU TO CLEAR YOUR SPACES OF THESE ENERGY FORMS--CONSTANTLY---I DO NOT TELL YOU TO NOT LOOK VERY CAREFULLY AT THEM. IT WAS WRITTEN THAT THE CONSCIOUSNESS OF EVIL WOULD REIGN UPON THIS WONDROUS PLACE BEFORE THE ENDING--SO BE IT!

I request that all ones reading these documents always take note of the date and hour, for you are receiving daily, if not hourly, input. In this instance, I will leave it to the editors to place this segment where deemed most valuable for I have kept this scribe from her appointed task far too long. Sir Tesla stands by and we Commanders have further input to the document.

We request that, even if unfinished, that this document be ready for book printing before week-end next from this one. Ones are in agonizing circumstance and in perishment every day that passes--and within these notes lay the focus and ability to pull together and get this matter of this last great plague under control. If you do your work well and create the apparatus in perfection, man need have no more great plagues--you will change your way of life-style--it will also mean a changing of perception of LOVE--there is LOVE which would bring no harm unto any and is in total giving---and that which you CLAIM to be LOVE in the guise of physical contact in a sexual manner which is self-pleasure and has naught to do with one another in definition. You continue to break all the laws of The Creation and call it man's "rights"---no, it simply brings about man's demise. I take no judgment of preference; I do take exception to "deliberate" actions which represent selfish lack of self-discipline hidden behind the facade of "love and rights". If someone of evil cut your throat and you are dying; would you turn and cut the throats of your cherished loved ones? That is what is occurring at every moment of your life these days---as I said long ago; ALL will be touched by this deadly plague--ALL.

Even if you are infected, every opportunity at reinfection only causes more contact, more bombardment on an already overtaxed system and more mutations of the retrovirus. May God be merciful and allow our task fulfillment in a timely manner. As a citizenry you must stand strong and demand life, do not follow in the path of the doomed lamb afore thee.

Please take a respite, Dharma, and then we shall return to the subject of the document. Thank you, chela, for sharing of your time, for these are most urgent and important interruptions. I am indeed grateful for the honest inquiries of such magnificent points and topics and bless those who speak that ALL might have explanation.

I leave this portion and move to stand-by. You will call when you are ready to resume, Dharma.

SALU, SALU, SALU   I AM HATONN TO CLEAR

CHAPTER 18

REC. #2, HATONN

FRIDAY, OCTOBER 20, 1989 11:15 A.M. YEAR 3, DAY 065

Hatonn present to resume input on the current journal. I have cause to be hesitant in information given forth for I fear I might misrepresent facts, or rather, that readers might assume incorrect endorsement of certain personalities who have, in actuality, only made a contribution in portion and are as divergent from truth in other portions as are the wild geese headed north for the summer. They have somewhat the same destination in mind but are truly flapping up great confusion in the face of already terminal confusion. I refer to any giving of credit to participants in the project of creating an apparatus for the cure of this plague at hand.

It would be good if you who are receiving this document, please use reasonable discretion in the subject matter. There are ones who give great assistance in the calling of public attention to the problem and "cover-up" but further their own belief in other areas of concern by integrating two differing subjects.

We are dealing with cosmic type, invisible frequency electromagnetic energy in the treatment and cure of disease. We are not into the business here of dealing with death rays, particle beams, enemy first strikes or warfare of any type. How or why you have a thing is only important to the extent that you isolate the cause so that it is not repeated and then recognize your precipitators and ultimately get a cure in the most rapid, efficient manner possible. If you become distracted into the international scalar beam possibilities you will remain distracted.

You must know of the systems which exist so that you can equally understand that the mechanism of cure is also valid. If a system works in one area of endeavor it can work in another if properly applied. Mr. Tesla could beam, wirelessly, electricity around the globe----that, friends, means that this of which we speak is most feasible. It does not need carry over into international warfare. As to warfare, if you get yourselves shelter for the old fashioned nuclear bomb devastation, you can survive the war to rise again. At this point in your myriad of problems, please do not borrow ones you cannot yet touch. First we creep, then we stumble, then walk and finally we run and ultimately we arrive at the goal. The problem faced here in the opposition of orthodox medical treatment is severe enough without borrowing the holocaust of perceived Russian invasion by Woodpecker beam systems; even if there were total truth to the accusation---that is not our subject at this point.

Yes, the retrovirus can be manipulated by pulsed beam systems---I have at my disposal a very good example. That in no way means that I am manipulating your viruses. Do not go foolishly forth making accusations which lock you into the inability to reconsider course. Accept these things for what they are, do not throw out the possibility but consider what you are about--right now you are "about" getting some operable apparatus to bring this great plague to a halt. Keep your direction and goal in placement one step at a time.

It is not even very unusual that you would find this type of treatment cast out as a fantasy. That is because the path of quackery has utilized the ploy of hocus pocus ad nauseam. Ones sit about in flowing robes and chant and meditate and "raise their vibrations", and thus and so. Well, as a matter of fact that is also valid. The problem is that it is most often a cop-out from truth and becomes silly foolishness. The mind can most surely heal and nothing will heal a thing without its cooperation and final "OK". The mind can more easily, than all your apparatus, create the necessary frequencies---however, you as a whole cannot accomplish that action. Do not fall into either trap--that of intentional death to a species by your "chosen" enemy nor the quirk that says you open your chakras to the tune of Yankee Doodle Dandy and all falls into perfection.

At this point in your evolution, you must have the apparatus in proper working manifestation and also the mind acceptance that it works---that individual master cellular system which functions from mind source--is your "other" terminal. You can kill every alien virus in the system and if the system doesn't know it, your entity will go forth and perish in spite of all you do.

You must understand that there is not only the ones who have perpetrated this blight, but there are also the ones who cannot "afford" to have the cure found. Dear ones, money--money--money! There are billions and billions of dollars involved in illness---there is hardly any material value in wellness.

A good progressive cancer patient is worth some $50,000 plus, walking around, to the surgery suite, to the chemical lab, to the radiation patrol and even on to the funeral parlors.

In your country alone, over 500,000 persons die every year of cancer and leukemias and now you have all this dandy AIDS "stuff". This represents a great bunch of money to certain vested interests. Stupendous and stupid investments in chemical drugs and medicines have been made and extremely huge incomes are resultant of the consumption of the modalities of treatment and consumption of these products and services. Medicines, drugs and so-called medical "science" have become just about your biggest consumer industry and your most hazardous to your individual well-being as a "patient".

You might ask, "But, AIDS can kill those medical people too, can't it? What will all those people do?" Well, you have the following situation involved. Those who are guilty, cover-up. Those who are educated in traditional ways, believe what they are taught until proven wrong---remember, the doctors, not too long past, put leeches on the body and bled people to heal them and didn't know what a germ was. Then, people believe what they want to believe until they can no longer even pretend the lie. It is a lot nicer to believe this AIDS will only get the so-called problem masses---the starving and ignorant in Africa, the hopeless ones on drugs, the homeless street people that society does not know what to do with, and then the socially unacceptable homosexual community. MAN REFUSES TO BELIEVE A THING OF

HORROR COULD ACTUALLY HAPPEN TO HIMSELF UNTIL HE IS STRUCK SQUARELY BETWEEN THE EYES WITH IT!

Further, the public demands rules and regulations and turns protection over, nay--demands it, into the hands of the government, etc. You demand the testing, testing of a thing for your protection, then demand the use of the item sooner than tested---then if it were badly tested, you sue. It is the story of the dog with its tail in its mouth--if it spins fast enough you cannot tell which end is which. It becomes obvious that everyone is terrified to "risk" anything. That, in itself, is horrendous for it leaves you at the mercy of the element who has figured that fact out to the best of their own advantage. Then you demand that same element solve the rest of your problems and then, in the end, you peer back and see that you have delivered yourselves to thine enemy's table, drawn and quartered and ready for their feasting.

Therefore, to accomplish that which must be accomplished, you must pull outside the orthodox entrapment, sponsor, support and ultimately fund your own project outside the sector of all the limits---take it outside your country if needs be---but get on with it. Taking pictures, quilts and posters in front of the White House won't do a thing, for the government can in no manner act quickly enough in this instance---you, friends, will do it yourselves or it will not be done. You must realize that you can focus your energy and funds into getting on with the job at hand. The red tape already established can delay you until the population is devastated. You are between a rock and a very hard place---you had better plan on moving one or the other out of the way---choose the one that gets the job done and not the one that only places more rocks within the roadway.

You do not need act in subversive manners nor destroy another's property--you simply need to focus the energyUand together create that which you need, without the negative distractions. You have willingly given away your freedom and now you must apply yourself positively and diligently to regain it. You do that through knowledge and acceptance of the truth--not through divided destruction and "fighting" but rather by united creation and pulling in unified togetherness. Therein lies the forgotten greatness of your country and your peoples in the wondrous melting-pot of mankind in the Americas. Must it require Armageddon to return brotherhood unto mankind? Look what happens in disaster---man helps his brother, he offers his own food, even unto possible death unto self does he rush in to pull another to safety----look most closely at this phenomenon for if you fail to return to this mode of living you have little to enjoy at any rate. Do you think the physicians inquired as to whether or not the mother, or the boy, who was trapped and near death on that freeway in San Francisco, might or might not have AIDS infection? A dead mother had to be dismembered to be moved to save the child and further, the child could only be freed by the amputation of the leg.

If you learn and accept the truth of your situation, clean up your act (literally), learn the facts--not the hogwash lies fed to you to keep the panic to a mere roar, and join together in that truth and contribution--you shall prevail. If you wait for another, or the government, or the medical profession, or the chemical drug houses to solve this problem, then I suggest you kiss it good-by now and save yourselves further discomfort. Except for this, there is no comfort in dying from any of the AIDS related diseases---hold it in your hearts. There is a solution! Will you choose to use it or will you choose to continue your journey in darkness and ignorance? It is solely up to you. GOD AWAITS WITH HAND EXTENDED UNTO YOU--YOU HAVE BUT TO REACH OUT PART-WAY FOR HE WILL ALWAYS WALK THE EXTRA MILE AND CARRY YOU IF NEED BE. OH YES, IT IS WELL PAST TIME TO BARGAIN WITH GOD; BUT, YOU HAD BETTER PLAN ON KEEPING YOUR END OF THE BARGAIN THIS TIME FOR YOU, AS MANKIND, HAVE COME TO THE "Y" IN THE ROAD. WHICH WAY WILL YOU GO?

Dharma, please take a short break to come back into focus on the subject at penning. I will discuss the harmonics of the laser when we return. All is light--ALL. How that light is applied and focused is all important.

I shall rejoin you briefly. Hatonn to stand-by

CHAPTER 19

REC. #3, HATONN

FRIDAY, OCTOBER 20, 1989 4:00 P.M. YEAR 3, DAY 065

GOD, THE CREATOR, IS LIGHT---THE INVISIBLE WHITE LIGHT OF THE UNDIVIDED AND UNCHANGING MAGNETIC UNIVERSE.

Hatonn present to continue. If I were to depart at this point, I have just stated it ALL. From the above comes all else. But we must dwell in perceptions and continual explanations that can tempt the mind into the acceptance of that which it, too, is. So, Dharma, you are long from finished with the lessons to be presented. Fortunately, however, if you know the "punch line" before the riddle is unfolded, then perception is so much more simple, indeed. For you it could be even more simple than you allow it to be for I do the thinking, so to speak, and you do the writing. You, on the other hand, must somehow ponder whether or not I speak truth and since you have no notion as to where to go for confirmation, you are stuck with the fatigue of "worry". So be it, little chela, so be it.

In God's Creation He limits all motion to that point in compression where invisible white light has been reached between the two visible yellows of flame in fission state. When a sun has become a true sphere its center has reached the white invisible still point in the spectrum where motion has ceased. Up to that very point the inward speed of compression has multiplied to its limit of 186,300 miles per second (in earth terminology, of course). At that point also, there is but one center of gravity. Until then there are two. White light is always invisible, for it is always still. It could not be white otherwise. Any motion, whatsoever, would be visible as yellow.

SO WHAT!

Well, you have just gotten the entirety of God, the universe and life and death, but I suppose I might point out a point or two for Dharma thinks I have forgotten AIDS. You will never solve the AIDS dilemma without the utilization of the frequencies produced by the harmonics of LIGHT!

The point I must emphasize is that when generoactivity has created a true sphere it also has created within it a white light of gravity to center it. (For you researchers, I have just made a most awesome statement.) It has also created its maximum speed and maximum temperature. It can go no farther. The Creator has consummated His Creation. He has given all He has to give. One half of His Law of Love has been fulfilled. Up to that point, earth friends, Mr. Einstein's equation of your 1905 fits to perfection. It fully accounts for the mathematics of life, BUT, not for death! The other half of the Law of Love must now be fulfilled. That which has been given must be equally regiven. The balanced rhythm of this universe must not be upset. For this reason that which has been must be repeated in reverse, to void that which has been, for neither life nor death can end or begin. They can only be repeated, and when they are repeated they do so through each other.

THEORIES ABOUT LIGHT

There are a couple of pretty good theories put forth by your scientists which can serve you sufficiently if you take a dimensional perception. One is that it is composed of particles; the other is that it is made of waves. You now know that, actually, both are correct. By the wave/particle duality of quantum mechanics, light can be regarded as both a wave and a particle--pulsed particles. Once the light is in motion it becomes "particles" or "harmonics" of the white light for it will either be increasing in frequency or decreasing in frequency---it is only "still" when in the invisible white state. It will be the harmonic frequencies of the various "rays" which will do your work for you.

LASER

In keeping with your love of your alphabet and acronyms, I would spell this out for your lesser interested parties. LASER means Light Amplification by Stimulated Emission of Radiation--no wonder you like your abbreviated version.

This is not totally correct in definition for a laser does not actually amplify light in the strict sense of your wording. It generates a particular kind of light and should in fact be termed an oscillator. It is also referred to as a quantum device since its action can be explained by the science of quantum mechanics; it is just unfortunate that you cannot find proper definition for that which you call quantum mechanics or quantum physics.

The important difference between ordinary light and light radiating from a laser is that the laser light is coherent. Each ray of light is of the same wavelength, or color, and is completely in phase with its neighbors, whereas the rays of ordinary light are scattered in all directions in varying colors and wave length. The energy of the light rays generated by the device is emitted in a varying sized thin beam which does not spread out, thus allowing it to be concentrated on a sharply defined point. The radiation can be made so intense that it will burn a hole in a steel plate of some thickness at a distance of several feet.

Radiant energy is propagated in the form of electromagnetic waves. A moving wave forms a series of crests and troughs, and the wavelength is defined as the distance between two adjacent crests or troughs. A wave has moved through a cycle when it has gone from crest to trough and back to crest again. The frequency of a wave is the number of individual cycles which are executed in one second.

Electromagnetic waves, including those of light, travel at the speed of approximately 186,300 miles per second. But you must change your concept into metric measure (which is still not completely accurate, but is used in scientific measurements). Therefore that value is given at 300,000,000 meters a second. Classification of all forms of radiant energy is carried out by a comparison of wavelengths, and a table can be set up forming a spectrum of wavelengths. The electromagnetic spectrum is so arranged that the longer wavelengths are at the bottom of the scale.

I am not going to give bunches of numbers for you who are researchers either know them or can look them up. We are efforting to establishment of scientific reasons whereby the scientific and medical community can accept, rather than discard as kooksville, the electromagnetic cure for your viral problems.

Only a very, very small fraction of the electromagnetic spectrum is visible to you as light. The lower region of that segment is visible as red light. The other as blue. I suppose to simplify things, I have to extend a bit farther into calculations so you understand how wavelengths are calculated. Your scientists created a measure called the angstrom unit, which is equal to 1/10,000,000,000 of a meter. This is abbreviated to the letter "A". The visible spectrum extends from 7,500 A (deep red) to 4,000 A (blue). The energy of radiation is proportional to its frequency, and the energy of each wave packet, or cycle, is called a quantum. This is measured by multiplying the frequency of the radiation by Planck's Constant.

Now, what is Planck's Constant? It is the quantum of action (symbol h). A universal constant. For any specified radiation, the magnitude of the energy emitted is given by the product "hv", where "v" is the frequency of the radiation in cycles per second. Your books give this constant as:

6.6256×10^{34} - kg meter^2 /sec. Plus or minus 0.0005.

NOW, I AM GOING TO TELL YOU THAT YOU ARE MOST FOOLISH IF YOU DO NOT RUN, BEG, BORROW OR KIDNAP BRUCE L. CATHIE FROM NEW ZEALAND--OR GO THERE. HE HAS CALCULATED A NEW CONSTANT WHICH FITS NEATLY INTO A SYSTEM BASED ON HIS UNIFIED GEOMETRIC EQUATIONS AND THEY TURN OUT TO BE CORRECT--A RARE THING INDEED. SO BE IT.

Dharma, let us stop for this day as it began before dawn for you. We draw closer to close of this document than you might assume. Mr. Tesla will be giving more of a lecture than great technical data so you shall find it most pleasant. Your public will have enough to ponder at one sitting.

I have great appreciation for your dedication this day and I take leave in such warm friendship and care. I am often filled to overflow with my affection for you dear ones who give endlessly to this wondrous time; my beloved students of these past months. Ah, the bonds can never be severed for we have grown together and shall ever remain as one. I salute you for your works well done.

Salu and good evening.

Hatonn to clear frequency, please.

CHAPTER 20

REC. #1 TESLA

SATURDAY, OCTOBER 21, 1989 7:00 A.M. YEAR 3, DAY 066

Hatonn present for brief comment and the morning quiz. That which you don't know can hurt you dearly.

How many of you connected the launching of the Delta for placement of a "military satellite" with the shuttle "probe"? Please keep your minds open for you are not told truth. The systems are getting a bit more sophisticated and if these "space" apparatus do not bear nuclear war weapons we can't touch them--hold it in your heart.

I further urge ones in the San Francisco Bay area of California to not settle into contentment in the assumption that "it is over for another hundred years or so", it is NOT. There is a very, very large shift due on the fault you label, Hayward. It was intentionally stabilized in order to not coincide with the quake just experienced. Further, this one did not relieve notable stress from the San Andreas; please don't simply return to sleep. My, you ones do like to tempt and gamble---back to the old ball game! So be it.

What does it require to keep you sleep-walkers awake? Well, let us get on with the work at hand. We shall endeavor to finish the document on this week-end for it is so timely. Therefore, I shall simply relinquish to our most respected teacher, Dr. Nikola Tesla, for he has waited patiently at stand-by for several days.

We have requested that he refra n from giving technical data regarding what you call "free energy" at this writing for our subject is so urgent and we are herein dealing with frequency and light. We shall get on to the other matter in proper sequence. Thank you, Dharma. You have spent many, many hours with Nikola but I shall be at hand if you have difficulty with communication. This is a good example of frequency integration, for you ones who think this type of communication is mystical or magic. Each energy who presents has a remarkably different frequency and some mesh more easily than do others. It requires frequency adjustments and can present a great deal of stress on the receiver until such time as perfect integration is achieved. Once achieved, however, it is quite easy at subsequent encounters.

NIKOLA TESLA

Tesla present and available for interrogation. I shall attempt to respond to queries which are already listed in prior meetings. Unfortunately, that which is requested predominantly, is not of this particular subject matter and I will acquiesce to solicitations to keep my theme within the boundaries of light---as you perceive it. All is light and it is most tragic to separate topics for if you have light you have already imposed all energy matters into the subject in point.

Since you already have available all you actually need to produce the apparatus under discussion in this document, I shall make an effort at bringing comfort between you who receive of this material and myself, that you might become contented and secure in my presence in this format.

I suppose my favorite lecture, while in your dimension, dealt with light perception as related to the most remarkable apparatus known to life--the eye. I shall bury a few "secrets" for the researchers who are assessing this material for missing keys to fulfill a given understanding. However, if you gather into a unit the proper workers, you have all you need. If each gives freely of his contribution, you can quickly and quite reasonably produce your equipment. I will discuss light, oscillations and electro-biological radiations and relevant material. Then I will get on with my wondrous appreciation of the eye if there is adequate time and the scribe does not desert me.

Your most valuable equipment, of course, will be Mr. Rife's fourth microscope (prismatic) of, approximately, your year 1935 along with apparatus allowing for the measuring of crystal "angles". And, of course, his fifth prismatic scope of approximately 1937 which narrowed the light field for slit ultra illumination. If you can reassemble those which have been secreted away you will be far advanced rather than having the necessity of constructing from start-up. I know they exist and are being worked on at this given moment.

You do not need concern yourselves to any great extent over the frequency apparatus for you can easily find far more sophisticated electronic equipment than was available for either Rife or Priore. But, always build upon the shoulders of others if their shoulders were headed in the right direction and their adjacent heads were screwed on properly.

In the start-up, however, you will need equipment that allows for extremely critical focused frequency, I suppose I am trying to say, refractometers, for accurate and wide-spectrum measuring of refraction indices.

Mr. Rife utilized a ray tube with mercury and neon--it would be more efficient if you would utilize, say, mercury and helium because of their octave opposition. Better yet would be bismuth and gammanon but you will find that a difficult combination to come by. Well, go with what is already available for it will be sufficient for this apparatus. Use your logical perceptions of proper frequencies as projected by Mr. Cathie.

You will not need a mammoth apparatus---always think in terms of "keep it most simple". Just as you can run electricity through every cell in the body by "passing it `through'" from one point to a completer point and cycle it back, the frequencies can be projected in like manner. I believe you will find Mr. Schroepfer will have some excellent input into that matter.

Just keep uppermost in mind that the physical plane (your perception limits of third dimension) is divided into sub-planes which differ from each other in one fundamental, namely vibration, which is characteristic of the density of the matter of each sub-plane. The sub-planes are generally designated as solids, liquids, gases and ethers of four differing grades. Actually there are additional grades, but this assumption will serve your purposes. The matter of the higher or finer levels interpenetrates those of the lower. Consequently, all physical objects, made up as they are of solids, liquids and gases, also have an etheric counterpart. This etheric counterpart, which all objects have regardless of size, is most important indeed.

All matter is in a state of vibration and your scientists have provided you with a scale of energy oscillations. I would, however, again request you consider Mr. Cathie's findings regarding this scale. Energy is measured in octaves, indicating the number of oscillations per second, and the medium through which such octaves are transported. This is why mercury is a most effective medium. The oscillations range from the first octave of two pentillion oscillations per second and are known as the X-rays.

SOUND

The first classification of energy is sound, extending from the fourth octave and the lowest audible note at 16 oscillations per second, to the fifteenth octave at 32,768 oscillations per second - the limit of human audibility. The medium through which this energy of "sound" travels may be solid, liquid or gaseous, and the propagation is performed by waves of condensation and rarefaction. Beyond the fifteenth octave, as audibility disappears, a range of oscillation comes into existence whose operations are defined as being in the "ultra gaseous" medium. This prevails up to the thirty-fifth octave and produces a form of energy known as "etheric sound".

Please consider this a bit of a primer. I suppose this is not such interesting reading as is a good novel but, dear friends, your species is at stake. Your medical profession must come into acceptance of this modality of treatment and they must do so most quickly. That means we must write some rather advanced items as well as quite primitive information so we can get a good scatter of information.

From the above described position, all sound slowly begins to change as much higher oscillations are approached, and on the forty-fifth octave the bombarding energy transforms and becomes manifest as "radiant energy", "heat", or "dark light". The travelling medium of this potency is known as the lowest or first "ether" and the character of its propagation is wave motion with molecular clash.

Now, push the oscillatory frequency per second further and at the forty-ninth octave the first, visibly, to appear occurs as red color. Your sense of sight enables you to appreciate the energy at this point, but although the organs of sight are the most highly specialized organs of the body and most closely associated with the central nervous system, their capacity is limited to a range of this one octave only.

As the analysis of the phenomena of light shows that the energy of this range of the oscillatory scale is transmitted by the medium of "ether", and unlike sound, is independent even of the medium of gas. A Radiometer, which is an instrument having vanes, mounted on a pivot in an airless chamber, shows rotation under its influence and the speed of its rotation is determined by the intensity of the light and the quality of its color. This experiment proves conclusively that Light is a force and a highly potent one, being able to register its effects across a vacuous space.

The source of all life and energy on the earth is of course the Sun, and its energy is conveyed to the earth by means of waves of light. Sunlight, on analysis, is shown to be a compound and composed of seven major prismatic colors, which always appear in the following order: Red, Orange, Yellow, Green, Blue, Indigo, Violet. These colors differ from each other in two ways, (1) the wave-length, which decreases from red to violet, and (2) the oscillatory frequency, which increases from red to violet.

For growth, all vegetable, animal and human bodies are dependent on sunlight for energy, which they are absorbing continually in the form of light and which they are radiating continually, though the manifestation is different. This takes place through the radio-active and radio-emanative organism or etheric counterpart of the dense physical body.

SPECTROSCOPY

Spectroscopy has shown that every element of the earth (over 92 now known) exhibits a preponderance of one or more of the prismatic colors and that the potency of an element depends on the potency of its color waves. It has been found that substances when burnt in a flame have the power of causing characteristic bright lines to appear in the spectrum; and that particular substances always cause the same lines to appear and always at the same location of the spectrum, regardless of the compound in which the metals were used or the great variety of chemical reactions in the various flames, or the immense difference in temperature of these flames.

This was true of the spectra obtained by a spark passing between electrodes made of these metals, and spectra obtained by a spark passing through tubes containing elements in a gaseous or attenuated condition. It was therefore unquestionably established that the bright lines of the spectrum are beams of light refracted to definite points in the graduated scale and are proof positive of the presence of the metals or elements in consideration. Each set of bright lines or refracted beams of light thus obtained represents the aggregation of wave-lengths, or in other words, the oscillatory rhythm associated with the composition or quality of that particular metal or element.

In the analysis of various elements it is found that, although some have many bright lines and others few, all show one or more lines predominant and usually one markedly so. This intensity of the lines and their concentration in a given position of the spectrum are the factors which determine the potency of an element and the range of wave-lengths in which it is most highly effective.

An element or metal heated thus before a spectroscope has had its molecular, atomic and electronic constituents so expanded that the oscillatory rhythm, being inherent in the element, can be appreciated visually by having it stepped up, by heat, to the forty-ninth octave. However, because of this integrity in the rhythm of the constituents of the metal, these oscillatory frequencies are detectable in octaves lower than the forty-ninth by instruments properly adapted for this purpose.

RADIESTHESIA INSTRUMENTS

By means of a specially adapted electric circuit, containing a bank of radio tubes, condensers, a resistance unit, etc, the oscillatory rhythm of the elements can be detected and their potency measured. This is especially significant when it is recalled that all foods and medicines, as well as the human body, are composed of definite element combinations, and therefore act in conformity with such color wave potencies, the aggregate of which gives each its characteristic oscillatory rhythm.

Using the above radio tube circuit, foods and medicines can be analyzed and identified as carrying potencies of color corresponding to definite portions of the spectrum. This is the key to Precision Therapy as will be discussed.

The human body is composed of elements, of which the principal ones are: Oxygen, Carbon, Hydrogen, Nitrogen, Calcium, Phosphorus, Sulphur, Iodine, Chlorine, Fluorine, Potassium, Iron, Magnesium, Silicon, and Sodium. These constituents, already shown to have distinctive and characteristic spectral bright lines of wave-lengths of light, would thus be representatives of the balance of energy existing in the body as light. The body, therefore, has certain oscillatory frequencies normally within it, each with a potency in direct ratio to the amount of the corresponding element present.

This is a most important fact which becomes apparent when it is known that, with the above electric circuit, the potency of these frequencies in the body can be measured and the excess or deficiency of the corresponding elements determined with accuracy. This is the key to Precision Diagnosis.

Different organs and tissues of the body having different chemical element preponderances, oscillate at different color wave potencies. In other words, the chemical activity in each organ or tissue, due to its normal characteristic element content, produces particular oscillatory frequencies which are maintained throughout health.

Oscillatory Rhythm and Electro-biological Radiations are synonymous terms. Any disproportion of the chemical elements of an organ or tissue, from whatever cause, would therefore have a marked effect on the balance of light energy in the organ. This would result in a changed oscillatory rhythm or electro-biological radiation from the organ.

A given disease condition that causes a particular disproportion of the chemical elements of an organ or tissue, with a particular disturbance of the balance of light, produces, as a natural consequence, an oscillatory rhythm or electro-biological radiation from the organ which is characteristic and indicative of that disease. Different disease conditions are associated with definite and characteristic tissue changes, macroscopical and microscopical. Coincidental and progressive chemical changes, registering as electro-biological radiations on the radio tube circuit, are equally characteristic and measurable.

Because of these facts the physician is able to detect disease in its incipiency and even in the etheric stage before macroscopic changes have proceeded to the point where symptoms are produced. This, of course, is of great importance in the field of preventive medicine.

Dharma, let us interrupt this dissertation for a rest break for this is a most lengthy composition and I am picking up great fatigue from your own frequency aura.

I would say, before we go farther, that it is time to allow Dr. Overholt to understand one of the reasons we had him peruse all the technical writings, some months ago, is to reassure this scribe that what we bring forth is most valid. It was a mammoth undertaking and our appreciation is great indeed.

I would further give appreciation to my contact in India who has already scribed this information from me. I am aware that it has been republished as recently as your spring of this year. It is most important that it be penned again in this document. Thank you for your patience and response to that need. It was first presented for a much different reason but as with all things, it is most applicable in this present undertaking. All things have a proper time and place of acceptance and understanding.

I shall stand aside while you have refreshment. I, in behalf of my colleagues here, extend our apologies at the length of these writings but they are most urgent and necessary.

Please notify me when you are available to resume.

NIKOLA

CHAPTER 21

REC. #2 TESLA

SATURDAY, OCTOBER 21, 1989 2:15 P.M. YEAR 3, DAY 066

Nikola to resume discussion.

I think it unnecessary to continue in-depth regarding this matter to any great extent. The point is that underlying conditions of disease show electro-biological radiations of their own that are separate and distinct from that of the particular infection associated with it. By utilizing various rates relating to various organs or specific areas of the anatomy, an area of inflammation or other malfunction can be isolated. A point of special interest is that owing to the anatomy of the large bowel, especially the Sigmoid portion, and also due to faulty elimination, theUaccumulation of toxins usually begins here, reaches the highest potential, and persists longer than in other parts of the body because there is ample area for extension and storage without production of symptoms due to pressure, irritation of nerves, etc.

I am not one who advocates colonics as a basic therapy as do many of your holistic practitioners. I found that utilizing a vibration frequency, suitable to the person being treated, would bring gentle and thorough results without discomfort or trauma. I have found that it is quite easy to adjust vibration frequencies to different organs of the body for parts have differing chemical element preponderances and therefore, oscillate to different color wave potencies. Any condition of disease is associated with a disproportion of the chemical elements of the body, with the attending disturbance of the color wave balance. You will find that many chiropractors will utilize these instruments whereby the medical profession, as a whole, considers them somewhat more quackery than judicial.

MEDICAL "DRUG" APPLICATION

It is most unfortunate that man cannot not have access to treatments based on logical progression rather than slash, burn and chemicalize at random in hopes of somehow salvaging a life, even if only partially. Don't misunderstand my intent in this dialogue, for there is most certainly need of trained and skilled surgeons and medical applications.

I will point out, however, that during the past 180 years or more, homeopathic students have organized a listing of remedies that are classified as to the capacity to counteract disease, and as to affinity for stimulating particular organs or tissues of the body. In selecting remedies by the radiaesthetic method, it was found that these tinctures and tablets not only coincided with the forgoing classifications but fell into groups corresponding to certain colors of the spectro-chrome diagram. Likewise, the more modern so-called "wonder drugs" (miracle drugs) also could be allocated to definite color positions on the diagram. I will not linger over the diagram at this time, but it is most feasible indeed.

Knowing the color correspondences of the remedies simplifies the matter of prescribing so that the balance of light energy in the body may be restored. After the causative factor has been removed or annihilated, there is always the need for restoration to proper function. In selecting the remedies for a given disorder, the one or more which could be expected to yield the maximum benefit to the patient would be those which, when matched against the patient's specimen, would reduce the congestion and infection potentials to zero and simultaneously raise the vitality potentials of the depressed organs to normal.

I have witnessed the utilization of ultra-sound in many modern instances, for instance, in pregnancy to visualize the infant in utero, without any damage whatsoever. It is most unfortunate, however, that your medical profession is so geared to monetary concerns and use of chemicals as designated by drug producers, that change is slow in coming. Much wondrous work goes forth in laboratories but it appears, as in my own life history, that that which is a true solution is barred from utilization, to a great extent. It further becomes obvious that if the retroviral infections afflicting your population are not halted quickly, your world population will be devastated--it is most distressing indeed.

I am bringing this portion, which may appear unrelated, but it is most important for the renewal process. Let me discuss it in relationship to a general malady which causes illness but is not life threatening, for example.

One beautiful part of ongoing diagnostic follow-up is that the remedy, even of maximum benefit, when administered to the patient accomplishes changes by degrees only. With each tonic or medication a certain percentage of the disease energy is neutralized and toxins eliminated. With subsequent check-ups new tonics are selected to fit the status existing at the time.

The road back to normal calls for aUreversal of the tendencies which brought about the condition, as well as the neutralization of the infection. The accomplishment of this objective requires the use of the principles of reinforcement or excitation at certain times and that of interference, retardation or impedance at other times. The important thing is to know when to use which. This is determined by checking, as example, the infra-green group and the ultra-green group of colors to see which are deficient, and which are in excess. While supplying the energy that reinforces the deficiencies and brings them to normal, the excess energies are simultaneously counter-balanced by interference or impedance. This holds true for any of the color designations.

The procedure is progressive and check-ups at intervals of a few days show the degree of progress, as well as indicating the "follow-up" remedy to meet the changed condition. Intermittent check-ups are essential because the effectiveness of the remedy, in tending to re-establish a balanced status, results in the patient out-growing it. In other words, these remedies of proven therapeutic value, prescribed according to this method of selection, mesh with the needs of the patient in a manner to promote elimination of toxins, to restore vitality to organs and tissues, and to re-establish gradually the balance of light energies in the body.

As you move into success with destruction of the viruses, you will not automatically have a whole and functioning body. You are going to have some very compromised people needing assistance in restoration to good health. Exposure to varying color beams from a spectra-chrome lamp, used directly on the patient, would be most beneficial, but a tonic corresponding to the same color sector, taken four times a day between lamp treatments, would greatly hasten recovery of health and vitality.

A point of interest as regards the various infections which attack the living organism is that while they are often composed of more than one kind of bacteria, the one most often complicating the picture is a virus. Then when you are faced with retrovirus infections you are compounding the problem. In general, a viral infection of general nature is relatively more persistent than the bacterial infection, which tends to melt away sooner under treatment, and yet, even they could be called "but nothing" compared to that which faces your species at present. You are going to end up with a body depleted of vitamins and minerals and the balance must be rapidly restored in order to disallow reentry of infection. Timely replacement of these items is mandatory.

I have rambled on at great length but it is most important to remember that a half dead patient free of virus is not a whole person. Although, with proper supportive treatment and cell enhancement therapy, recovery can be amazingly rapid.

I would suggest that another marvelous thinker be brought into your circle of colleagues, Trevor James Constable. Mr. Constable has done excellent, and proven effective, work in radionics. You should look closely, indeed, into geometries of radionics and cosmic life pulses. Well, I feel it inappropriate at this writing, to go into CYMATICS, which is practical healing with the use of sound, or psychokinetics. All, in the summation, utilize light frequencies which at appropriate vibration produce both sound and color.

It is, in summation, most urgent that you move forward with your research in the cure of AIDS for it is even more deadly than you have surmised. It is further, obvious that you will never get the cure established if you await governmental or professional medical community intervention in a timely manner. Your bureaucracy is much too leviathan to allow a timely solution.

This information should be scattered throughout the most involved communities as quickly as possible and further, the populace who feel themselves safe, must be given the facts. If your private sector will pull together, you can accomplish your goal. I repeat, you have ones who already have the abilities necessary; you simply need to pull them together into a working, full-time unit.

Obviously this will require funding; however, since this plague affects every man, woman and child on your planet I would foresee that as this is made known, ones will contribute the necessary support.

I would request that ones be urged to purchase this material rather than simply passing it around, for the writers of this material are dedicated to great contribution to the rapid realization of a cure---every day, henceforth, is most precious.

Dharma, I have made a decision to not impose further upon your patience nor on the good nature of the readers of this journal. I shall give my dissertation on the wonders of the eye at a later, and more suitable, time. I am often accused of eccentricity in these dimensions as well as when I tinkered within yours. Ah, if I could grant a few wishes, I would give the quality with which I was gifted, that of constructing my machines and apparatus in two dimensions. I could literally project and construct in the invisible fourth and experience the workings thereof without the cumbersome density of the three dimensional plane. But that, too, shall come unto you ones sooner than you might perceive.

I will take leave now, that you might move on with your activities. I am in great appreciation, Dharma. I trust my contribution will be of some value, although, I am confident my contribution will be much greater in other areas of creation and invention. You ones must never overlook my bladeless pump for it serves in so many various manners. I look forward, with great pleasure, to working again with you and my colleagues.

I am most cordially yours in friendship,

EPILOG

REC. #1 HATONN

MONDAY, OCTOBER 23, 1989 7:45 A.M. YEAR 3, DAY 068

Hatonn present, and I believe that we might pretty much finish the document on AIDS this day. There will be others as we move along in "time" but this is sufficient for man to come into understanding.

As instructions to the compiling I request the following.

As an Epilog (in placement), I will herein give appreciation to Paul Andrew (we may not utilize his full name for several reasons, not the least of which is that we shall not have him tracked back to his mother). You will please insert the following statement afore the taped transcription and continue it as the final chapter, as such.

****

ACKNOWLEDGEMENT OF HONOR

GIVEN FORTH THIS DAY OF OCTOBER, 23, 1989, YEAR 3, DAY 068

* * * * *

In the entanglements of the physical life journey there are many "unsung heroes" who come forth and during their lifetime they are ignored, persecuted, ridiculed and at best, misunderstood. These ones come in sequence out of an acceptable time element and are projected among a band of humanity not ready for acceptance of the gifts they bear. All who scan these pages will know of one or more such individuals. They come in all sizes and shapes, colors and creeds. Most do their appointed task and depart; man never realizing the treasure borne forth and cast aside through ignorance.

One such gift unto you ones, was a man whom we shall only label "PAUL ANDREW" for it is most critical that this personage not be traced back to birth source at this time.

He efforted diligently at "fitting into" your world. He never succeeded, and having come forth to alert others in a timely manner, he departed your plane at the age of twenty-five years.

There were two people who never fully heard his pleading cry and others who, in their mindless way, drove him in torment. Earth man will learn truth of his actions and stand responsible for their egotistical errors, for once upon your plane an energy is locked into the same format of existence as are all others.

Paul, even in the smallness of his years, and in spite of the bombardment of negative fulfillment, came forth with what he called his theory of DIMENSIONAL LIFE. The version printed herein is not his polished document which was put to tape some six weeks later, but must suffice in concept for the tape was damaged greatly. Ah, some of you will say: "But that is my theory also, so what is new within its message?" He put it forth as a gift and perhaps you have not yet taken your stand for truth and understanding of that truth; no more and no less.

Paul was birthed into human format on July 30, 1959, in your American city of Salt Lake City in the State of Utah. All who knew him also knew he was not from your place. He physically departed on March 22, 1985 from Bakersfield, California. His entity departed your plane on March 31, 1985 from the area north of Glendale, in your Los Angeles County, California. I give these coordinates that those who recognize of my words will have confirmation.

He served well, he serves well presently and shall be allowed to bring forth his works in absentia of that afore mentioned entity and through other conduit. Man must learn that his perception of life-streams is incorrect and come into understanding of endless life and mind.

As in STAR TREK, those who will be coming forth to assist you from the fourth dimension are only more advanced than are you, little brothers, they are not Gods and are not one WITH God, until they have completed their individual life-stream "tours of duty", if you will. I shall not dwell further on the subject at this time. I shall again, in other documents, give further credit to this young energy who made the ultimate contribution.

There are two human energies he respected and loved above all others; his mother and one labeled Dr. Andrew J. Golombos. The mother began to understand, the good doctor failed to come from his self-appointed lofty position upon the pedestal to ever see the "Bruno" or "Halley" he had within his grasp. Woe be unto man who fails to recognize of the gifts. Dr. Golombos has wondrous gifts to offer but in his self-appointed definitions separating egotism and egoism--he missed--the definitions are correct, the actions most incorrect. He could, however, sort out all of your technical problems in a very short time-span. If his humility ever matches the projection of his words, he shall be included. He can be easily located in the area of Los Angeles, California.

The earth father of Paul Andrew shall also remain unnamed. His contributions were ones of pain and denial, greed and ignorance. He, himself, is a physician who has yet been unable to heal himself. Honor shall be given when honor is earned and merited.

I do give honor to the step-father who understood finally, albeit too late for the human being, he has since contributed in unlimited measure unto our cooperation. I must also leave this one unlabeled for security reasons--this message is for him to receive at this time.

I will further request that those who know of whom I speak, look within and without for you are missing thy opportunities of greatness.

For you who seek truth, do not fall away for the petition is always heard and if requested in truth of desire and in honor, ye shall be given it.

IN RESPECTFUL HONOR UNTO MY SON, PAUL, I PLACE MY SEAL OF TRUTH AND SORROW THAT MAN IS SO BLINDED IN HIS DARK IGNORANCE.

I AM ATON

******

PAUL/DIMENSIONAL LIFE

SATURDAY, OCTOBER 14, 1989 12:29 P.M. YEAR 3, DAY 056

TRANSCRIPTION OF AUDIO TAPE MADE JUST PRIOR TO PAUL'S DEATH

TAPED JAN. 19, 1985, 12:45 P.M.
PAUL'S DEATH: MARCH 22, 1985

SUBJECT: DIMENSIONAL LIFE

PAUL'S THEORY OF DIMENSIONAL LIFE

What is the idea of dimensional life? For an explanation of "what it is" I must go into a few details leading into the theory.

The first is the concept of dimensional universes. We live in and understand the "zeroith" universe. If we were living within an atom this would be the negative-one universe (-1), and if we departed the "zeroith" (0) universe, or we stepped outside of our universe, we would step into the positive-one (+1) universe. Then we would look upon our universe, or the zero (0) universe as an atom. It would then appear, but I have no way of knowing how far in either or both directions the stream flows, i.e., - 1,2,3,4, etc. and + 1,2,3,4, etc.

Being within the current universe which is represented by the zero (0) status, I cannot say for sure if these other dimensions actually exist, but for definition sake, I will say that we live in the zeroith universe. Therefore, if we could move within an atom we would have to say we are in the -1 universe. Therefore, if we move outside our universe we would of necessity be in a positive, say (+1), universe. Briefly, that is a simplistic concept of dimensional universes.

Let's now say you have a line going from negative through to ours, the zero, and on into the positive dimensions of the universe. Now what if somehow one could step outside of that line--then you would be in the cosmos-or free in an etheric state of existence within the cosmos--free of universal restrictions. Now this is but a concept which, to my knowledge, cannot be proven.

The next point I would bring to your attention is what is called the theory of evolution--certainly an old concept which has been under great contradiction and controversy as presented by Charles Darwin. This theory, if I understand it correctly, is that basically man came from the higher apes, the apes from lower species and on down the line through the fishes and back to the tiny one-celled life forms.

But, if you move farther backward, so to speak, you move downward through perceived life form and into molecular reactions, or chemical reactions.

Keeping in mind my concept of dimensional universes, and further, keeping in mind Mr. Darwin's theory of evolution, at least if the above understanding is correct, we would, of necessity, move into what I call, dimensional life. This concept, if correct, becomes the theory of dimensional life.

Now, the idea is essentially the following: Let us say, that we--as man--live in the zero universe. That is, right now the human species is consuming energy and consuming resources. We are expanding our growth. As we expand our growth, our needs for more resources, our needs for more energy also grows.

As man continues to grow he will eventually leave the planet Earth, move to other planets and will begin utilizing the energy and resources of other planets, firstly from those in our particular solar system. Man, then left to his own devices, will continue to grow and exhaust the resources in these new environments so he would need look to other sources for man continues to expand without thought to eventual destiny or extinction.

It is feasible that man, in his movement into the solar system, will expand and eventually begin to pull other solar systems together, but man shows, so far, that as he now incarnates he would just continue to use the resources in exploitation. In any case, man will expand ultimately to the limits of our galaxy and then at some time in the perceived future, provided man continues to grow and expand, the energies and resources in our own galaxy will not be enough. Therefore, at that time, man would of necessity move on out into other galaxies.

Let's say that the +1 universe looks upon galaxies as atoms, and let's say that man finds it most beneficial to connect galaxies together for the best utilization of the energies and resources of the whole. Now, if you were moved into the positive one universe looking down at the atoms, what you would then see would simply be represented as chemical reactions with those atoms ("galaxies").

If you look in the opposing direction, you would say that there is a sharp line between the zero universe in which we live, and the negative-one universe, which are atoms. It could be that in the positive-one universe the entire of the galaxies could represent one atom--or, from higher dimensions the entire of the galaxies may appear to be as one atom. My knowledge is not great enough to know wherein lays these sharp lines of demarcation.

I have already given you the image that if we begin pulling galaxies together--then, you would have a chemical reaction within the positive universe. If, however, the entire of the galaxies are represented as one atom then man could still continue to expand until, relatively speaking, he expands to the limits of the universe as his current perception would recognize such and move into a higher "universe" whereby he has more energy and resource with which to function. This obviously would not be in a physical format as we can recognize of it in our current structure.

At that time he may find it more appropriate to connect universes together, at which time you would perceive chemical reactions within that prior positive-one universe. Where those sharp lines between these existence frames actually is, I simply don't know. You can look at universes, galaxies, solar systems or groupings of atoms as if they are only one atom.

Let us look at this zero universe where man now stands and assume we have worked our way upward into the positive-one universe. Well, actually, let us move in the other direction and look at the realm of the negative universe, or the atoms.

Now, Mr. Darwin indicates that we first had chemical reactions, followed by one-celled animals, on into fish and plants, then animals, and then finally, man. What is all this leading to? After coming this far, I hope that you will understand my meaning when I say, "What is man? What are you? What am I?". Each one of us represents an entire civilization of some type of life-form, or social structure composed of trillions of living entities functioning in our perceived negative-one universe---obviously controlled and placed into order of function by our system already in a representative higher universe.

Your body, yourself, may be an entire civilization composed of hundreds of billions, actually trillions, of living entities residing in the negative-one universe controlled by a central "computer" or "God" who is obviously "self", for if the controlling mechanism--you--breaks down, you then have chaos within that negative-one universe--your body.

So, what is dimensional life? Dimensional life may be this; that you have living entities in one dimension that build social and organized structures large enough to become a single, living entity in the next higher dimension. As those single entities in the next higher dimension, multiply and grow, they in turn build yet another structure which ultimately becomes cohesive and functions as a unit and moves onward and upward. This is never ending for there is no limit to the universes themselves for universal realms are infinite. Essentially dimensional life is the progression of life-stream into ever higher and more orderly compilation of units into ONE whole. From the zero status this cannot be proven, but at some point I believe man will be able to have knowledge from the higher life planes and this will be brought into our knowledge and be proven.

What I conceive here, I would like to think of as the theory of dimensional life. Right now, in my frustration, I have no way to prove this theory and certainly few would entertain my opinion for there are many much more learned men than myself and I probably would not be heard. I know there is a fragment, an essence of energy that can only progress, for having progressed (evolved into higher form) it cannot move backwards for that is the law of progression. In this instance it would have to be said that this my "hypothesis" of dimensional life for a "theory" actually needs more scientific proof to be acceptable and I have no means for its proving.

When I think about it, and the more I think about it, the more I am convinced it is real and it is correct and orderly. Then, I get completely in awe of ones who have been able to utilize the concepts of living things upon which to base their physical constructions.

When I look at a mosquito, a fly--even those tiny little gnats, those little tiny gnats that fly around in circles about an inch in diameter and get in your ears and sit there and go whring, whring, whring and go in your eyes and ears and bug hell out of you, I have to look at them and think how wonderful it is that they can actually fly. I think about ones like Wilber and Orville Wright and how intelligent they really must have been to actually figure out how to fly. I think, "what an achievement that is!" and then I really wonder how can a mosquito fly? How could it know how to fly?

Then I realize that man could not build a mosquito. Man could not build a fly. With all our current technology, high as it may be, we still could not build a mosquito---something that small that could fly--well, we could not build a mosquito!

So what did? Something did! I conclude that what did are living entities beginning in the negative-one universe. The same flow stream of living entities that built you and me. Boy, it amazes me when I look at a fly. It amazes me when I look at bugs because I think, "What in hell built them?"--something built them and it sure as hell can't be by accident.

Something actually built me--something built you and it sure as hell was not by accident.

Let's look into the other direction where man expands. We start connecting up, let us say galaxies. Before we realize it, we find ourselves in an ocean of galaxies. Or, if you are in the positive-one universe looking back (or down), you can see an ocean of atoms and maybe some molecules which have begun to connect. You realize that YOU can connect those atoms and before you know it you find out, damn, you can actually move that civilization through this ocean. Well, there would be God's one-celled animal in the positive-one universe, which is not shabby.

Well, you can use your own imagination from there. When man starts building two-celled animals, or two-celled societal structures and three, and then four and then a thousand and a million . . . .

I look at a mosquito and think of a helicopter, I look at a bird and I think of an airplane and I think, "Where is technology?" Man developed technology for helicopters and airplanes, but who developed technology to build mosquitos and birds? Oh my--well, let us look now at another evolution.

Let us look at Wilber and Orville's first powered airplane, the very first powered flight. Look at the evolution of aircraft from its inception through its growth, up to today. On a parallel to that you could look at the first "thing" that flew, it probably was not a mosquito--who knows, maybe a bird or a fish--one that could flop its wings and remain out of water, whatever it was --- look at the very first one. Well, there is type evolvement or natural selection whereby each developed, or was orderly constructed, to efficiently function and continues to evolve to be more adapted and efficient.

Could not man have a similar parallel growth? Could he not grow up and beyond the limits of this dimensional restraint and into higher dimensions of life-type existence?

Well, you have my theory for dimensional life. Yet, I have no proof nor do I think I am the first to have this concept but neither have I found it written elsewhere. Therefore, I can only draw conclusions which I feel to be logical and I therefore believe this is valid.

If I am correct, this could lead to many, many other things. If it is true that these living entities actually are in a negative universe awaiting expansion, growth and order then perhaps we can communicate with them on a frequency or vibrational level. And secondly, perhaps they are seeking a way of evolvement themselves, in their primitive aspect, and by our being higher, but composed of them, perhaps we can show them how to build even better than ourselves, you know, maybe we could lead them a little better---I truly believe that each cell--each atom--has a frequency and by use of that particular sound or light frequency we can actually communicate and structure order out of any chaos in the mechanism.

In looking at man who is now above the negative-one universe it appears we have not progressed in proper fashion, therefore, by communicating with that negative-one universe we see that if we do not utilize technology--let us compare our brain to that of a computer, if we don't use the computer wisely we will be overrun with chaos from that negative-one body which can produce equally negative balance over into our current living universe which I refer to as the zero state.

The computers, the mind, seem to get larger and larger and appear smarter and smarter. This also leads further-- and I would like to think about something else which has just come into my thoughts.

When the computers which man is now utilizing, become so powerful in themselves, that computers can make their own decision solely on their own, it will affect the destination of man himself because man will have given up his rightful place in the order of progression. Right there, at that time, you essentially have produced another "living" entity or "being" composed of matter and brought it into a higher existence.

When the time comes, as it appears it will, that computers make the decision for the species---however developed, that they gather data that makes the decisions instead of man, that will be a very important point in time. When I think about it, that is starting to happen right now, because already reliance is placed on computers which come up with facts that are critical and vital to the human species. I can see that relatively speaking, in the near future worldwide computers could be making decisions for the functioning of the entire human species.

Well, looking on the other hand, if you and I are separate civilizations in the negative-one universe then it seems to me that the brain may be one of these computers, in concept. If so, then this idea can carry further into a magnificent brain (computer of energy) which controls all of us and each of us.

Looking at the idea of dimensional life, I have come across other things which seem to make sense, to me at least. When you look at our civilization growing and expanding, you can use your imaginations and imagine unlimited things when you parallel it with the negative-one universe. When you look at the negative-one universe from the aspect of the zero universe, you can thereby imagine what our zero universe must look like from the aspect of the positive universes.

The idea of dimensional life may very well be important in guiding the human species in the future by acknowledging and understanding the living entities in the negative universe and seeing how they have progressed. We can do two things, we can help them to progress better and at the same time, we can learn from their progression in order or chaos and likewise adjust.

Let me restate this idea. By acknowledging and understanding, well, first you would have to prove that the negative-one universe living entities actually exist in such a universe; and further, prove that we are a product of their work---a product of the architects and engineers of that universe. Now, by understanding and observing their progress, it can be most beneficial to our progress as a human race, for it is the end result of how those atoms, molecules and cells function which ultimately reflects how we function on the whole. Therefore, it could be most beneficial to our overall societal structure.

Further, by monitoring their progress, we can actually help them correct their course if it is in disorder, and give them the resources they need. We could find out what their structural and societal needs are and help them and in so-doing, they will help build us and our higher potential can even better assist us as we move onward into positive higher dimensional living. We could go forward with a lot fewer mistakes if we would just pay attention.

I guess this pretty much concludes my ideas of dimensional life as I have called it. I do hope that someday it is proved so that if some day it does become a theory of dimensional life, I believe it will be very powerful for the advancement of knowledge, the advancement of the human species and the betterment of all life.

There are two people, if they had not existed and I had not had the input from either one of these two people, there would absolutely be no way I could have developed. One is Andrew J. Golombos and the other Charles Darwin, though I disagree with his final conclusions.

There are thousands of people that I wish to give gratitude and I thank all of the people that have helped me. I could read off a list, but I would first have to make the list, and it would probably contain too many to list, therefore I just give my appreciation to all who came before me.

I thank everyone who has given me input and I am most grateful. I also wish to add that up to this point, I have not written on this matter. At this point, I give anyone rights to expand on this subject with only one request, that they give me some credit for these ideas. If it is, however, not an original idea and therefore belongs to another, such as Dr. Golombos, then I withdraw all rights; no one shall use these ideas unless they are truly mine.

I further require that the writings be only for the betterment of mankind and that they in no way hinder or damage anyone else's property.

This concludes the taped message, but I see that I have quite a bit more available tape. Since I will be studying this subject I will leave the space for addition of material.

There is one other thing right now. When I was thinking of putting this on tape for people to hear, I could only think about what if I am wrong---what if people say, "Paul, you are a fool!" Well, what I have put down is only a concept which I have developed from much input and that is all it is. I correlate it with painting a picture. Say, I painted a picture of the Golden Gate Bridge, well, that would be a picture of a very "real" thing that exists, ok, and say I made duplicates of that picture and gave it to others. Well, I have painted this picture and I give it likewise as a gift, as represents my perception.

On the other hand, let's say I sat down and I dipped my paint brush in a randomly picked color to begin and I sloshed the paint around on the canvas and then dipped my brush in different colors, never cleaning the brush and just did a mish-mash---which a lot of artists do these days (and they sell pictures like that). Well, this may be one of those mish-mashes or a piece of art--in either case it is my idea and I give it as an idea for I cannot prove it in any case.

Again, thank you for hearing me.

Good-by---

Hello again, a couple of additional points, please.

Every time I spoke of molecular reactions, I wish to include crystal growth. I did mean molecular reactions but must include the growth of crystals.

When I spoke of the computer intelligence, etc., what I mean is not individuals in that civilization but the civilization itself as a whole, as to action and direction.

The third point I would like to add is; as to the rights of anyone writing a book on this subject---that is open and I hope that someone does so--I very much hope that someone does. As to the use of the material; anyone can utilize the substance as long as it does not hinder or damage the property of any other individual.

Also, on the subject of the computers; don't misunderstand--I do not think the computers as machines will ever have power to function independently, it will be through consistent and ongoing interactions with individuals; so in that sense they will never have total power to make decisions, but I think you understand my meaning.

I would like to leave you with one question in mind to think about. When you look at plants and animals; say you look at a bug and ponder over how it came to be---could this be the solution, could the idea of dimensional life really be valid? Please inquire of yourself the next time you look closely at a living organism such as a plant or animal.

Again, thank you.

END OF TRANSCRIPTION

****

ABOUT THE AUTHORS

WALTER RUSSELL

This was such a great, great man. I shall give no technical data for if you know of whom we speak, you can look up the documentation; if you know not, it would mean naught. We will simply repeat his "Foreword" from his book "THE SECRET OF LIGHT" for that was his work most relative to this document at hand. Given in your year, 1947.

"Jesus said, `GOD IS LIGHT,' and no man of that day knew what He meant. The day is now here when all men must know what Jesus meant when He said `GOD IS LIGHT.'

"For within the secret of Light is vast knowledge yet unrevealed to man. Light is all there is; it is all we have to deal with, but we do not yet know what it is. The purpose of this message is to *tell* what it is.

"Today's civilization has advanced far in knowing HOW to deal with matter but we do not know WHAT matter is, nor the WHY of it. Nor do we know what energy, electricity, magnetism, gravitation and radiation are. Nor do we know the structure of the elemental atoms nor the gyroscopic principle which determines that structure. Nor are we aware of the fact that this is a two-way continuous universe of balance in all effects of motion and not a one-way discontinuous universe. Nor have we even yet heard of or suspected the most important of all principles in physics, THE VOIDANCE PRINCIPLE and the mirrors and lenses of space which are the cause of illusion in all moving things.

"Nor do we even consider the entire material electric universe to be the illusion which it is; there being no reality to it whatsoever.

"Nor have we the slightest inkling of the cause of curvature of space, nor the voidance of that curvature in planes of zero curvature at wave field boundaries. No one now knows how it is that crystals get their various shapes. It will amaze the world to know that those shapes of crystals are determined in space by the shapes of the wave fields which bound the various elemental structures.

"Nor have we the slightest conception of what constitutes the life principle, nor the principle of growth, nor the simultaneous unfoldment-refoldment principle which repeats all patterns in Nature sequentially and records and voids them as they are repeated. Nor are we aware of that recording principle by means of which the Creator carries forth the sum totals of every sequential cycle in His unfolding and refolding universe unto the very end of its manifestations upon one planet and its beginning on a new one.

"Nor are we dynamically aware of the souls and seeds of things. These roots of universal repetition are now but metaphysical abstractions to religion and physical guesswork to science.

"Within the secret of Light is the answer to all of these heretofore unanswered questions, and many more, which the ages have not yet solved. This revelation of the nature of Light will be the inheritance of man in this coming New Age of greater comprehension. Its unfoldment will prove the existence of God by methods and standards acceptable to science and religion alike. It will lay a spiritual foundation under the present material one of science.

"The two greatest elements in civilization, religion and science, will thus find unity in marriage of the two. Likewise, human relationships will become more balanced because of greater knowledge of universal law which lies behind all of the processes which light uses to interweave the patterned forms of this electric wave universe.

"There is no department of life which will not be vitally affected by this new knowledge of the nature of Light, from the university to the laboratory, from government to industry, and from nation to nation.

"I therefore give it to you with all of its clarity as I myself have become aware of it from behind the scenes of this cosmic cinema of light illusions which is our universe."

WALTER RUSSELL

And for all his wondrous works in the philosophies, arts, atomic sciences, all his connections with famous personages and from all his accolades from the highest human sources; his one desire was to bring enlightened truth to his fellowman and KNOW GOD! So be it.

* * * * *

NIKOLA TESLA

Born in Yugoslavia, Nikola Tesla landed in New York in 1884 at the age of 28, one of thousands of immigrants to come from Europe to the United States that year. He arrived with four pennies in his pocket--and his mind bursting with brilliant ideas which would stun the scientific community, introduce humanity to the true potential of energy, and light up the world.

In comparison to his contemporary, Thomas Edison, Nikola Tesla's name is not well known. Yet it should be, for without his scientific breakthroughs and inventions, our modern world would be very much different than it is. You would have Edison's light bulb, but only people living within a mile or two of a power station would be able to use it. For it was Tesla's development of alternating current generators, transformers, and motors that overcame the immense limitations of Edison's direct current systems and made the long-distance transmission of electricity practical. It was truly Tesla's genius which lit up the world -- not just homes for the wealthy.

Nor was Tesla's genius limited to just this one accomplishment, as staggering as it was. He invented the Tesla coil, which is still used widely today in radio and television sets and other electronic devices. He pioneered the use of remote control. He produced better turbines than anyone else. He created artificial lightning. He harnessed the electrical potential of Niagara Falls--a stupendous feat in his time.

In 1900, twenty years before the first commercial radio broadcast, he attempted to construct a mammoth tower on Long Island to broadcast not only radio and television waves, but also other electromagnetic energies. It was a grand scheme which would have revolutionized the shape of modern life even more than his other projects--but it fell through when financial support was withdrawn.

At the height of his success, Tesla maintained an elaborate laboratory in New York. From time to time, he opened the doors of the lab to the public and gave demonstrations about the nature of electricity and the new developments he was working on. The demonstrations were often quite spectacular, with Tesla calmly sending electric current through his body to light up an incandescent tube he was holding. (This is not terribly unlike the method that will ultimately cure AIDS.) The lab itself contained many innovations which were never commercially exploited. None of his lights or motors, for example, were connected to the power source by wires. Instead, a single loop ran around the four walls, near the ceiling. This loop was continually electrified, and from it all of Tesla's lamps and motors "somehow" drew their power.

As impressive as Tesla's inventions and innovations, however, are the breakthroughs he made in the scientific understanding of the principles of electricity. More than anyone else before him or since, Tesla comprehended electricity. He knew how it behaved and what could be expected of it, not just from observing electrical phenomena, but also from directly perceiving, intuitively, the archetypal patterns of electricity.

It was this understanding of the nature of electricity which allowed Tesla to recognize the value of alternating current and how to make it practical--at a time when other scientists had pronounced it nothing more than a scientific curiosity, with no useable merit. It was likewise this profound understanding and insight which drove Tesla to conduct a series of experiments in Colorado Springs, where he proved the existence of terrestrial stationary waves--proved that the earth's atmosphere is electrically charged and can carry electromagnetic waves from any given point to any other point on the earth's surface. He considered this discovery the most important of his career, and put it to a practical test, broadcasting electricity through the air without wires and lighting lamps twenty-five miles distant with it. Even scientists of today do not understand fully the significance of these particular discoveries.

Sadly, many of Tesla's best ideas never went beyond the experimental stage. A world occupied with its mundane concerns could not appreciate the treasures of Tesla's transcendental thinking while he was alive, and did not adequately support his work financially. Indeed, late in life, Tesla had hardly any funds to finance his scientific investigations. Yet he kept pursuing new understandings, even though the majority of his insights would not be applied.

ONE OF HIS MOST SPECTACULAR IDEAS, THOUGH, DID GAIN A CERTAIN AMOUNT OF ATTENTION. HE DEVELOPED A "DEATH RAY" WHICH WAS CAPABLE OF SENDING DESTRUCTION THROUGH THE AIR UP TO DISTANCES OF 250 MILES. RECOGNIZING THE DEADLY POTENTIAL OF SUCH A DEVICE, HOWEVER, AND THE INABILITY OF MODERN GOVERNMENTS TO USE IT WISELY, HE KEPT THE PRINCIPLES BEHIND IT A SECRET.

Tesla ALSO EXPERIMENTED EXTENSIVELY WITH THE PRINCIPLES OF RESONANCE, which is the capacity of the energies of one physical object to vibrate in step with the vibratory patterns of another object or force. He comprehended these principles well enough to be able to create artificial earthquakes with a most tiny machine--and claimed he had the knowledge to split the earth like an apple. Today, many scientists are trying to rediscover, in their work, the principles of resonance which Tesla explored in his--but did not receive the support to develop.

In fact, a great mystique has been generated in certain circles about this man and his discoveries. Russian scientists are trying to duplicate his "death ray" as are the American scientists. However, without proper understanding there is a very likely chance they will simply "split the earth like an apple" for they have no notion as to how to control that with which they toy--alas, to the possible destruction of the recognized world and the species of man.

Few are able to reproduce his thinking and understanding of scientific principles and those who come close practice at greed and self-proclamation of inventor status just as took place in his lifetime.

This is worth musing on. In the long run, it is not the inventions and the breakthroughs which should be considered the greatest contributions Tesla made to mankind, as spectacular and as important as they were. MR. TESLA REQUESTS THAT THE NEXT PORTION BE EMPHASIZED: FAR MORE IMPORTANT WAS THE STYLE HE SET FOR SCIENTIFIC THINKING AND DISCOVERY. TESLA WAS TRULY AN EXAMPLE OF ENLIGHTENED GENIUS, AND SET A LEVEL OF BRILLIANCE THAT SHOULD BE THE MODEL TO WHICH ALL SCIENTISTS, GENIUSES, AND INTELLIGENT PEOPLE STRIVE.

TO TESLA, THINKING WAS A PROCESS WHICH BRIDGED THE OBJECTIVE, PHYSICAL WORLD WITH SEVERAL SUBTLE REALISMS, WHERE IDEAS AND CONCEPTS EXIST ALMOST LIKE FISH IN AN OCEAN, WAITING TO BE CAUGHT BY THE INQUIRING HUMAN MIND. HE WAS NOT SATISFIED WITH SPECULATING ABOUT IDEAS AND THEORIES; HE PUSHED BEYOND SPECULATION AND LEARNED TO DEAL WITH IDEAS AND THOUGHTS IN THEIR OWN REALM, WHERE THEY CAN BE FULLY PERCEIVED.

IN OTHER WORDS, TESLA USED THE MIND TO LINK HEAVEN WITH EARTH. HE IS CERTAINLY NOT THE FIRST PERSON EVER TO DO THIS, BUT MOST OTHER GENIUSES WHO DO LEARN TO BRING HEAVEN TO EARTH DO IT IN RELIGIOUS, PHILOSOPHICAL, OR CREATIVE WAYS. WHILE THEIR CONTRIBUTIONS ARE VALUABLE, THEY ARE ALMOST ALWAYS COUCHED IN VAGUE WORDS AND INTANGIBLE FEELINGS ABOUT LIFE, LIGHT, AND BEAUTY. TESLA, BY CONTRAST, FOCUSED THE IDEAS OF THE MIND TOWARD SCIENTIFIC DISCOVERY. HE TRANSLATED HIS IDEAS NOT INTO VAGUE PRECEPTS AND LOVELY THOUGHTS, BUT INTO TURBINES, LIGHTING SYSTEMS, BROADCASTING TOWERS, AND ELECTRICAL MACHINERY. IN HIS HANDS, THE LIGHT OF HEAVEN LITERALLY BECAME LIGHT ON EARTH.

I, Hatonn, would like to make one last comment in this vein of thought. Mankind always takes unto himself these thoughts and projections and changes them somehow to suit self. In Mr. Tesla's case, it does not work so efficiently as in the religious world, for if you do not utilize Mr. Tesla's concepts quite purely, you will not be producing a functioning machine. You must know, however, that his ideas have been stolen from inception through this day.

His favorite offering to questioners regarding his brilliance was simply attributed to Isaac Newton: "IF I HAVE SEEN FARTHER, IT IS BECAUSE I HAVE STOOD ON THE SHOULDERS OF GIANTS."

* * * * *

COMMANDER ANTHIOSE XANDEAU ASHTAR

COMMANDER GYEORGOS CERES HATONN

We will not linger over lengthy definition of our history for those bothersome tidbits are covered in prior material and has little value here other than as distractions. Please suffice it to say that we are most valid and come in love and truth, sent at this time in service of the higher Source. It is with great gratitude that we participate and have humble appreciation for being graciously received.

As we move ahead, we trust you will come into your trust of our presence for you have been misled for so long a period of sequence that you have forgotten your source. As we bring forth corrections to your myths which have become distorted through the cycles of your "perceived" time it will be necessary that we have established absolute truth of both our presence and content of information.

We most eagerly look forward to the approximate sharing of this transition of "time" and "space" change. It is toward a true brotherhood of mankind in all dimensions that we now are coming into your physical consciousness that you may be prepared for our physical visitation.

The purposes of these messages is one of making acquaintance in friendship and to give assistance through a most critical and trial laden portion of your evolution. It is, further, to allow you to recognize that the dimensions of experience are only "different" not invalid. We are most valid indeed, there is nothing mystical nor magical about our invisible presence---all works within the laws of universal physics; we are simply higher dimensional beings who are more advanced in technology and knowledge of The Creation and Universal Truth.

In love and appreciation for your kind audience, I now bring this document to a close. May God be gentle and merciful upon you dear brothers as you journey through this most difficult time sequence. We are at ready and prepared to assist if you but petition in equal peace and integrity.

COMMANDERS ASHTAR AND HATONN TO SIGN-OFF PLEASE. THANK YOU.

Transmission concluded 10:31 A.M., October 23, 1989, Day 068, Year 03.

OUT

INFORMATION

To obtain the Strecker Video Tape send $32.00 directly to:

Robert Strecker, M.D.
The Strecker Group
1216 Wilshire Blvd
Los Angeles, California 90017

For information regarding the Aids Medication mentioned on Page 6 telephone the office of:

Earl Rice M.D.
From California 1-800-262-0212
From outside California 1-800-523-8795